SUPER EASY
WOOD PELLET GRILL &
SMOKER COOKBOOK

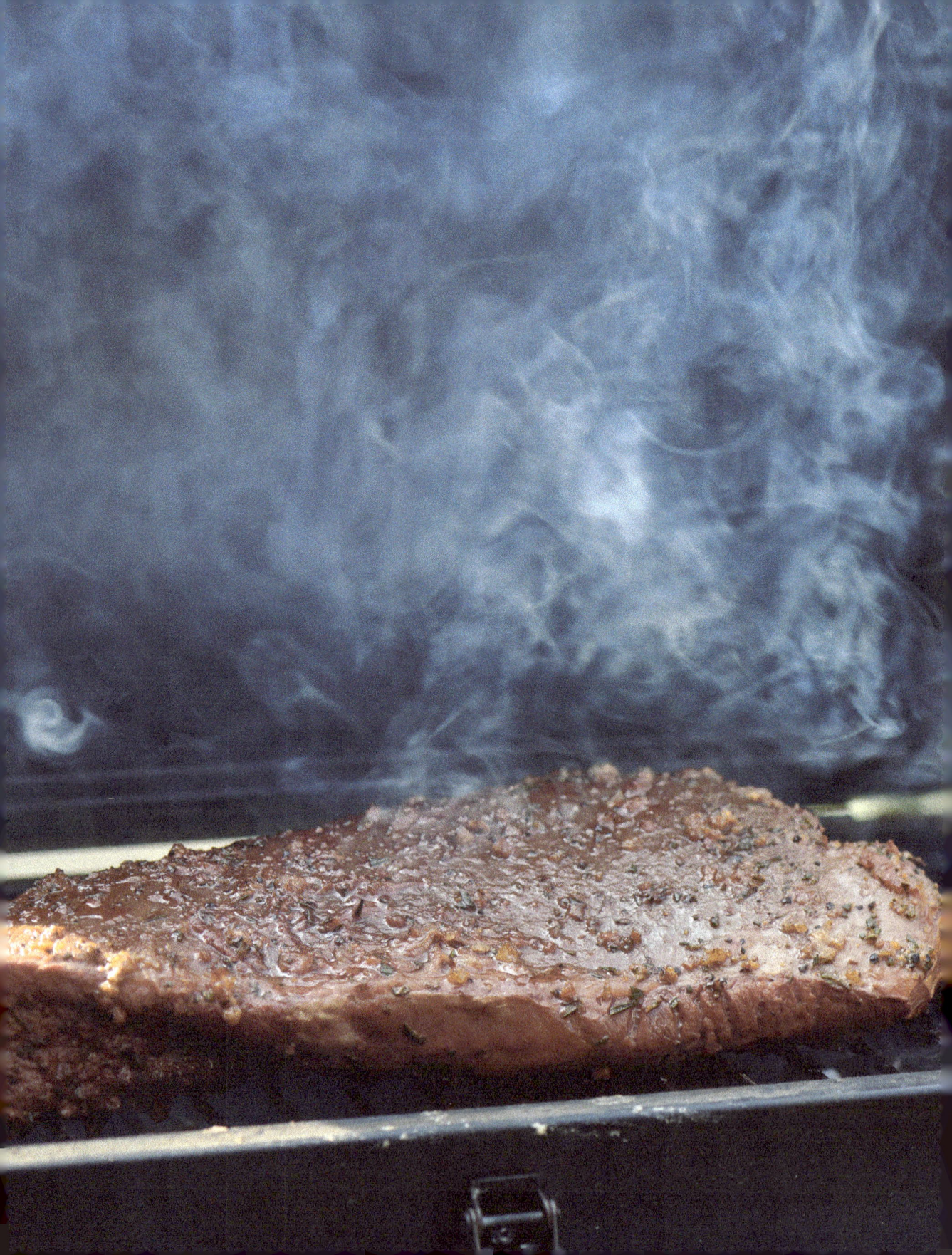

SUPER EASY

WOOD PELLET GRILL &

SMOKER COOKBOOK

55 Effortless, Full-Flavor Recipes

ANDREW KOSTER

PHOTOGRAPHY BY DARREN MUIR

R

ROCKRIDGE
PRESS

For all the barbecue restaurants,

restaurant employees, and

caterers who have been affected

by the COVID-19 pandemic.

→ CONTENTS

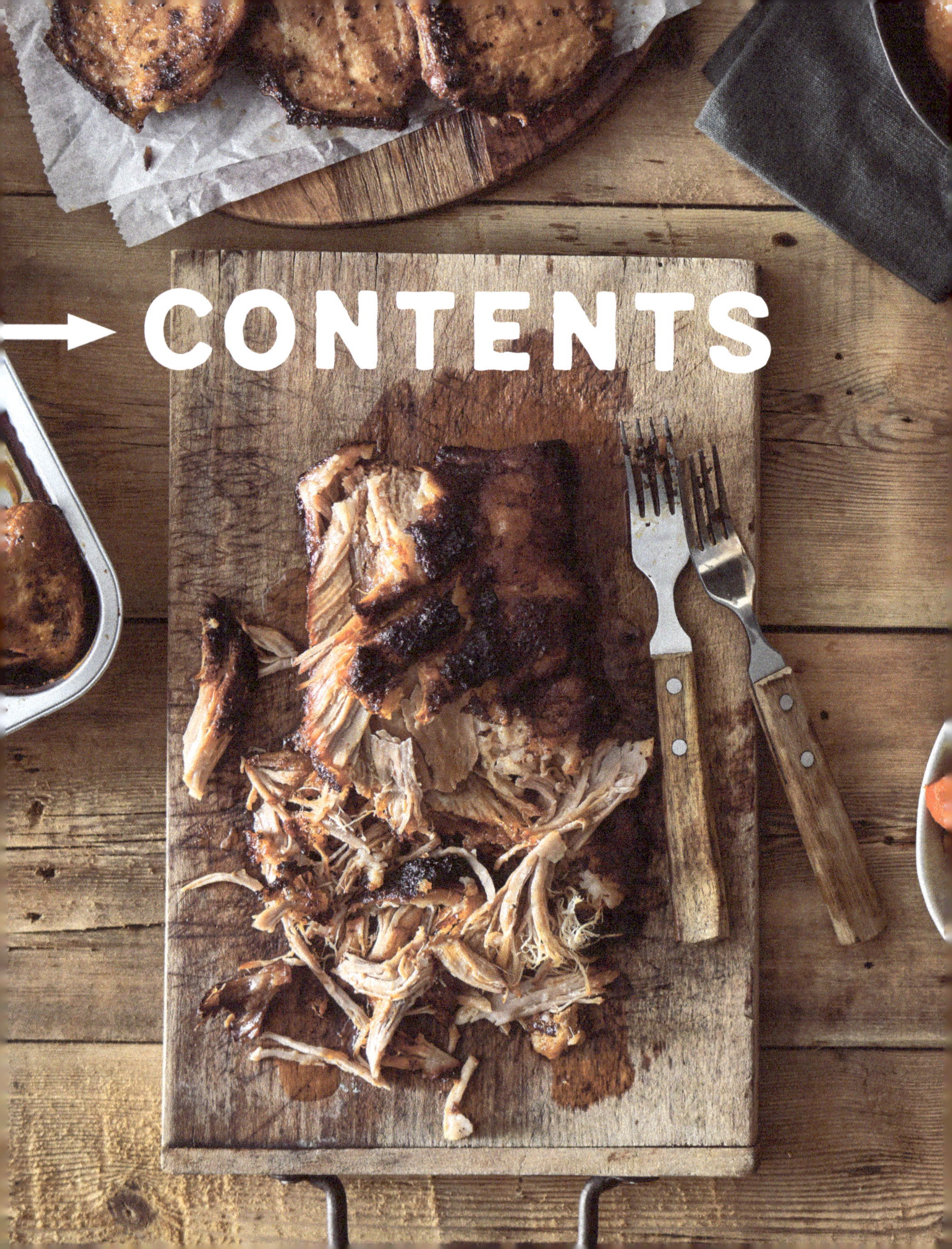

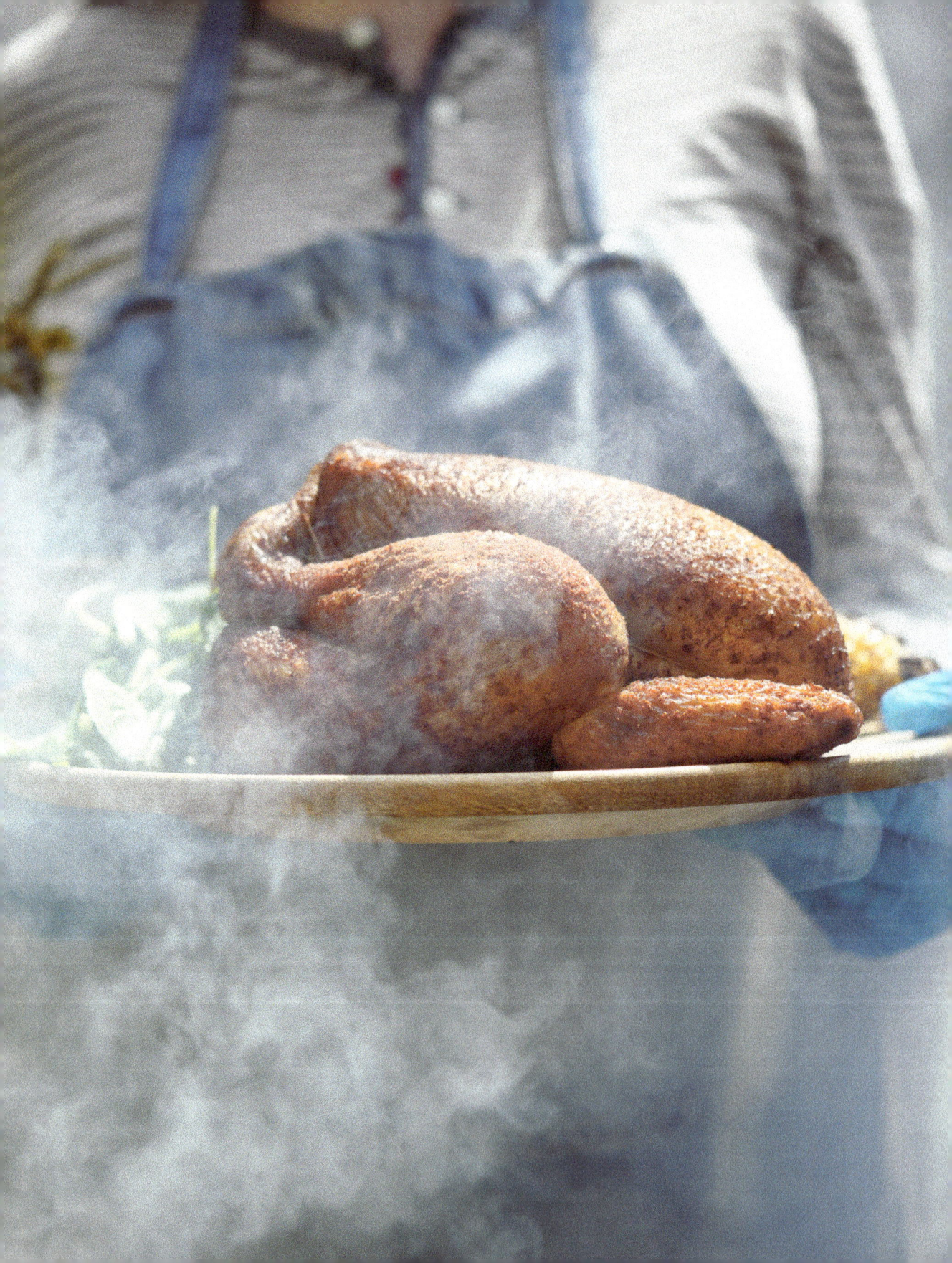

INTRODUCTION

I began my journey in pellet grilling far earlier than most people. My father, George Koster, was one of the first employees at Traeger Industries to work in pellet grills and, with the exception of Joe Traeger, is the longest-tenured employee in the business. Growing up, our sports teams were sponsored by Traeger, and pellet-grilled chicken was a staple at local high school sporting events. I would frequently work small jobs at the old barn in Mt. Angel, Oregon, where Traeger grills were manufactured for about 25 years. Being around the grills so much allowed me to learn a lot about them. Before graduating from high school, I knew all of the main components of a pellet grill and how they made the machine work. Watching both my mom and dad cook on the multiple grills they owned over the years showed me the basics of how to barbecue.

After graduating from college, I went to work for Traeger. I was the customer service manager there for five years, before holding the same position at Pit Boss and at Louisiana Grills for another year. All the things I had learned over the years helped me to teach others. I am currently in product development at Dansons, the makers of Pit Boss, Louisiana Grills, and Country Smokers. In this role I have made many significant contributions toward building the best pellet grills on the market, most notably the Pit Boss Pro and Platinum Series. I also just filed my first patent!

Now, as the primary chef of my household, my cooking style predominantly revolves around the grill, and I rarely come inside to cook. I love to try a wide variety of techniques and recipes and am always extremely confident in both the process and the result because of the versatility of the pellet grill. Being a part of the grilling industry helped. I was frequently asked how to cook things, and the only way to learn was to do it myself.

Joe Traeger invented the pellet grill with just that in mind. The ability to use your grill with confidence is the premise behind the product. No more fires. No more dried-out or burnt food. Taking the system he was already using for heating and repurposing and optimizing it, Joe created the ultimate wood-fired cooking machine.

The ease of use of the pellet grill is its greatest feature, and that is what I will focus on in this book. All pellet grills afford their users a great amount of versatility with a generous learning curve. You can practice, learn your grill, and learn to cook without ruining your meal.

Throughout this book, you will find simple recipes that will give you the fundamentals for using your grill and a starting point for creating your own masterpieces, resulting in amazing meals for you and your loved ones. All recipes call for a limited number of ingredients and little prep time. We're going to let the grill do the work.

Along with being simple to execute, the recipes in this book take full advantage of what your grill has to offer. Most of us think of "low and slow" cook times as "long and tedious" when we think of barbecue. Though we will definitely cover that process, most recipes are time efficient. After going through this book, you will have simple, delicious recipes for your next party, tailgate, or Tuesday night. Whether it's roasting, barbecuing, or searing, you are going to do it all!

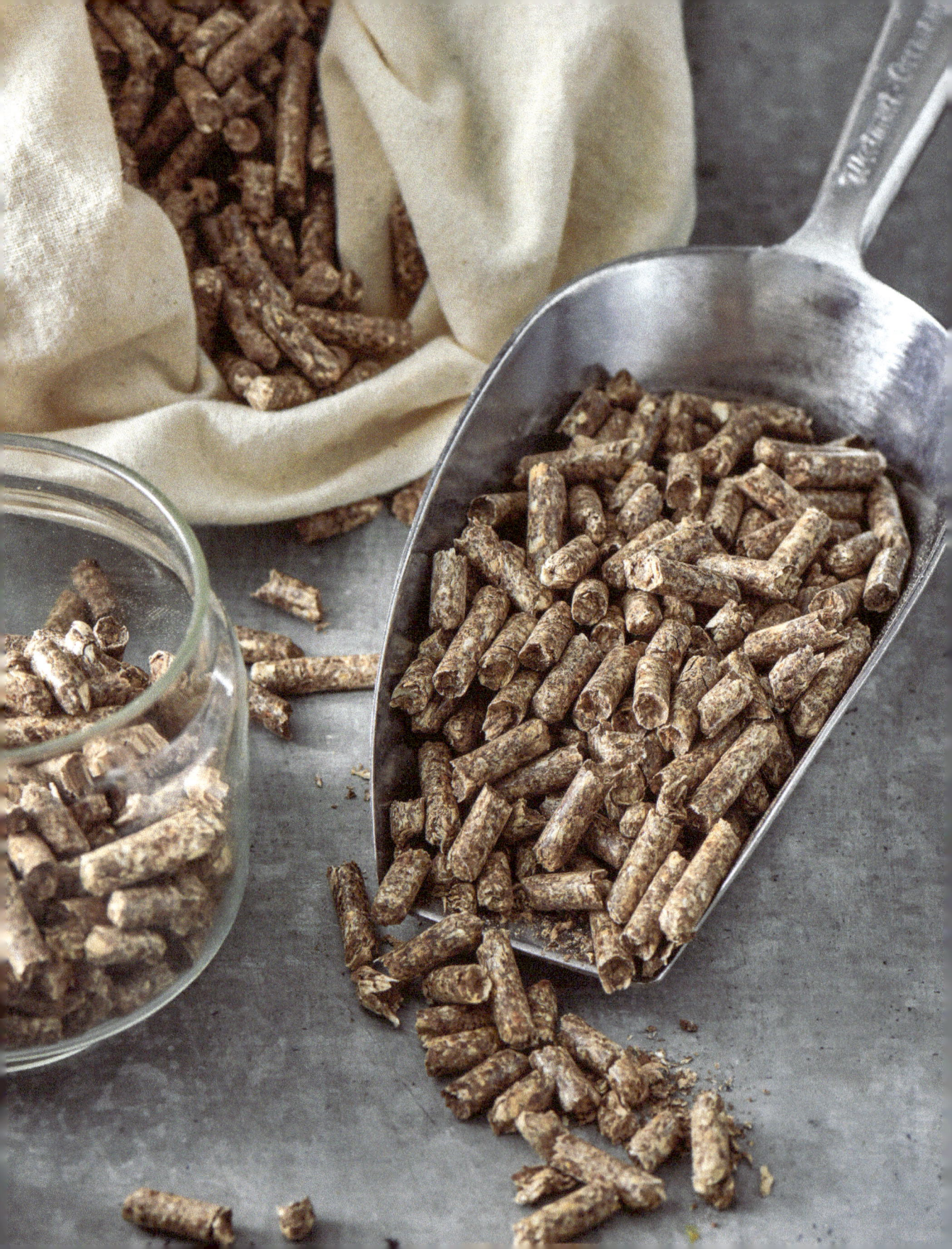

chapter 01

SMOKING WITH YOUR WOOD PELLET GRILL

The pellet grill is a relatively basic machine that uses an auger feed system in tandem with induced air to maintain heat and smoke inside the grill chamber. Though the premise is basic, understanding how the grill works will help you conquer any food on your menu.

Throughout this chapter I will go over the ins and outs of a pellet grill and all the tools that you can use to master it. By learning about the grill itself, the cooking process will be simplified exponentially.

WHY WE LOVE THE WOOD PELLET GRILL

There are many reasons to love your pellet grill. From convenience to cleanliness to versatility, the pellet grill has become the most attractive grill in the industry, and there is good reason for that.

As someone who grew up with the pellet grill, it is one of my greatest enjoyments to explore other grills and see how they compare. It wasn't until I was in my thirties that I began using other types of grills. Though there are upsides, like achieving specific flavors or ultimate temperatures, I often find myself trying to make them mimic my pellet grills.

No Messy Charcoal

We have all been there, getting ready to prep the perfect meal on the grill, only to come back into the house looking, and smelling, like a chimney sweep from the 19th century. The pellet grill eliminates this without compromising flavor. By using the grill's digitally-controlled feed system, with an auto-start feature included with all of today's grills, all you have to do is set the grill to smoke and walk away. The grill will light itself and you can go inside to prep your meal, smelling of that expensive designer fragrance you love instead of smoke and charcoal.

Precision Temperature Control

The pellet grill comes with a giant upside over the competition. It uses a controller to deliver the precise amount of fuel and induced air to get you to whatever your desired temperature setting is. The digital controllers on today's grills use this technology to maintain an average temperature with minimal variations, consistently creating smoke.

Today's controllers come in a few different varieties, but each has the same goal in mind—to maintain a steady temperature, while also creating smoke.

Clean Burning with Little Ash

When pellet grills started to gain mainstream popularity in the early 2010s, I was the customer service manager for Traeger, the world's largest pellet grill company at the time. One of the more frequent questions received from new customers was, "Why does the inside of my new, black grill look blue?" The answer was in the clean burn of the pellet grill.

The burning in a pellet grill is extremely efficient. This is why the smoke appears blue, unlike the dirty, creosote-y smoke that you are used to from other grills or smokers. This also means minimal ash cleanup. You are able to use a pellet grill multiple times without the need to clean out the unburned fuel.

Versatility

The pellet grill is, hands down, the most versatile grill on the market. It can do with ease what traditional grills could only dream of doing. From smoking to searing and everything in between, the pellet grill can do it. Just set the grill to the desired temperature and get to cooking the way you know you can.

Pellet grills can smoke, bake, braise, barbecue, grill, roast, and sear. Brands like Pit Boss, Louisiana Grills, and Weber even give you the ability to char grill over an open flame.

HOW IT WORKS

The pellet grill is a rather simple system. An auger-driven pellet feed along with induced air work to maintain a fire created either by an igniter or manually by the user.

Based on wood pellet stoves, the original pellet grills would turn the auger on and off to maintain either a heat range or set temperature, with a constant fan speed. While this is still the predominant functionality of many of today's grills, some have begun using DC, multispeed motors, and fans. This accomplishes much of the same thing, but allows for more precise temperatures and different ways of inducing smoke.

Pellet Hopper

Every pellet grill has a pellet hopper designed to deliver pellets to the auger. Though these hoppers come in different designs and sizes, they all have the same purpose. Today's hoppers can be massive. Some of the larger grills have hoppers with upward of 45 pounds of capacity. Many newer grills have dumps as well, allowing you to dump your pellets out to protect them from moisture or to switch woods.

Auger

The auger is what delivers the pellet fuel to the fire. The grill's attached motor slowly turns the auger and moves the pellets through it. Auger sizes and pitches, as well as the speed of the motor, can vary. These differences are typically found in grills of different sizes because bigger grills need to move more pellets.

Firepot

The firepot is where all the action is. Pellets are delivered to the firepot and ignited. There are specifically designed holes in the firepot that are made to deliver air to the fire. Firepots are designed with functionality in mind. Any adjustment to the firepot, no matter how little, can have huge effects on how the grill functions. Smaller grills will typically have smaller firepots and fewer holes.

Igniter

A grill being able to light itself is extremely convenient, and today most pellet grills come with this feature. Pellet grills use an igniter in the firepot to light the pellets. The igniter uses the most electricity of all the parts, but it is only on for a short time. After the pellets are lit, the fire is self-sustaining. Some igniters are also used as a safety feature, turning back on for extreme drops or low temperatures. If a fire goes out in a pellet grill, it is a potential hazard. Pellets can pile up in the auger,

and restarting the grill when this happens can start a very large fire. Turning the igniter on in adverse situations prevents that pileup of pellets from happening.

Cooking Grate

Cooking grates for pellet grills come in a variety of types. Most grills come standard with porcelain-coated steel or cast-iron grates. Some grills, primarily high-end units, come with stainless steel grates.

Many of today's grills also come with multiple levels of grate racks. Additional racks give you the ability to cook a large amount of food at once. Cooking grates are removable, so if one isn't needed or gets in the way, just take it out.

Drain Pan

Because you are not cooking over a direct flame on a pellet grill, it is necessary to drain the grease from the grill somehow. To do this, a drain pan is used below the cooking grates. Drain pans come in different shapes and sizes, but most function the same. A tilted drain pan catches the grease as it is released from the food and funnels it to a bucket or pan outside the cooking chamber.

Induction Fan

Without airflow, there is no fire. The fire needs oxygen, which is forced into the firepot with the induction fan. Different grills use different fans that are optimized to give your grill's fire adequate air. Larger grills need more airflow to handle the increased amount of fuel being delivered to the fire.

Controller

The controller is the brains of the grill. It communicates with a temperature probe inside the grill to determine how much fuel and air to deliver to the firepot in relation to the set temperature and chamber temperature.

There are currently two types of controllers that dominate the market: digital cycle controllers and PID controllers. Both do the same thing but go about it differently. The digital controller replaced the standard three position switches in the 2000s. It relies on the smoke cycle (p-setting) to maintain the set temperature and typically creates more smoke. PID controllers are newer to the industry and use enhanced technology to send pellets to the auger more frequently, in smaller quantities, which results in more precise temperatures.

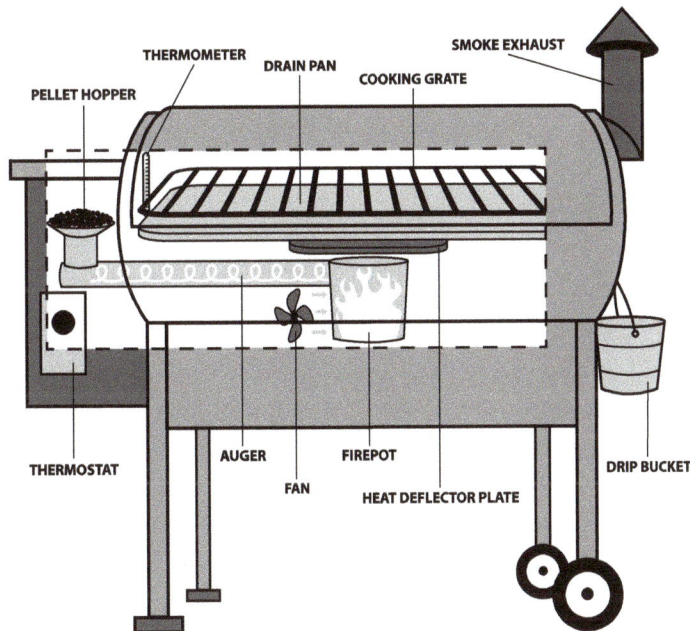

THERMOMETER DRAIN PAN SMOKE EXHAUST COOKING GRATE PELLET HOPPER THERMOSTAT AUGER FAN FIREPOT HEAT DEFLECTOR PLATE DRIP BUCKET

THE HIGHS AND LOWS OF THE
WOOD PELLET GRILL

The temperature range for most pellet grills is 180°F to 500°F, though there are some that offer ranges outside of that, like the 600°F of Louisiana Grills or Traeger's 165°F.

Pellet grills use convection to heat the chamber because the drain pan blocks the direct flame. This is what allows you to cook your food while almost never burning or drying it out. Because of this, there is also little need to turn your food during the cooking process—it is being heated throughout on all sides, rather than by a direct heat source like a traditional grill.

The smoke temperature is relative to how little fuel you can provide the firepot without completely losing fire. Pellet grills always need to have a fire going, even on the smoke setting. New innovations have come about to improve the temperature range of the pellet grill, reaching extreme highs and lows that previously could only be achieved in other types of grills, creating the ultimate grilling experience. Hybrid gas/pellet grills give consumers the best of both worlds. Companies like Pit Boss and Cuisinart have led the way with these grills that have two fuel sources, one gas and one pellet. These grills have the ability to get to the extreme high temperatures of a gas grill.

Companies like Oklahoma Joe's, Louisiana Grills, and Pit Boss use sear plates to char grill with a pellet grill. These units have the ability to open the area directly over the firepot, giving the griller a 1,000-degree flame. Weber has also opened their pellet grills' drain area completely, similar to their gas grills, giving their users a full searing area.

Cold smoker attachments and smoke tubes can give you the extreme low temperatures that you need for smoking cheeses, nuts, and other foods that require lower temperatures.

ACCESSORIES AND TOOLS

To become the ultimate pellet griller, you need some basic tools. Luckily, you don't need many. Here I've listed some of the most necessary, but the great thing is that a lot of these items come with your grill.

Instant-Read Thermometer

If you only buy one tool that I suggest in this section, this is it. Many pellet grills today come with meat probes built in, but in my opinion, nothing beats an instant-read thermometer. The most important component in creating the best grilled meats is temperature. Take your meat off too early or too late and you're likely to ruin dinner.

Wi-Fi Controller or Thermometer

Wi-Fi-integrated grills have to be the biggest game changer of the last decade. I love the ability to see what is going on in my grill when I'm not there. Companies like Weber and FireBoard make amazing thermometers that work in tandem with user-friendly apps to create a great grilling experience.

Wi-Fi has also found its way into the grill itself, giving users full control of their grill while also tracking grill and probe temperatures. Brands like Green Mountain and MAK led the way in this technology, and companies like Traeger and Pit Boss soon followed suit.

Cast-Iron Grill Grates

Cast-iron grill grates are a great addition to any pellet grill and are an upgrade to steel grates. Cast iron holds heat far more effectively and helps give you those awesome grill marks you're looking for. Brands like Pit Boss and Louisiana Grills offer cast-iron grill grates out of the box on most models.

Smoke Tubes

I have to admit, I used to be a major critic of smoke tubes. I thought, "Why put a smoker into a smoker?" I was totally wrong. Not only do smoke tubes give you more traditional smoke flavor, they can be used to turn your grill into a cold smoker. I regularly use my A-MAZE-N smoke tube when smoking everything from ribs to cheese.

Cold Smoker

Cold smokers are a great way to explore another avenue of cooking with your pellet grill, and they also give you increased space to cook. Cold smokers or smoker cabinets attach to the grill where the chimney typically goes and give users a secondary chamber that is significantly cooler than the main grill chamber. Use a cold smoker with your grill set to smoke and cold smoke cheese or fish.

Grill Pan or Basket

Grill pans and baskets are necessary for cooking foods that could fall through the grill grates. Veggies and the like scream for a grill basket. Using grill pans and baskets allows you to take full advantage of the grill. Foods that you might not typically think to put on the grill are suddenly full of that wood-fired flavor.

Grill Cover

Protect your investment! Most pellet grills are built to last for years, and a grill cover helps you keep its finish protected. Beyond just keeping the outside of your grill nice, a cover keeps water away from your pellets. Moisture-affected pellets swell and disintegrate. To anyone who has had this issue in their grill before, I've been there and feel your pain.

FUEL FOR THE FIRE: FOOD-GRADE WOOD PELLETS

The pellet grill relies on food-grade wood pellets for its functionality. These small pellets, about the size of a pencil eraser, are made from sawdust or hardwood fiber and held together by pressure. The process of creating the pellets packs about 10,000 pounds of pressure into each small pellet, and the heat generated allows the wood's natural adhesives to help bind the pellets.

These hardwood pellets come packed with different flavor profiles. Pellets are made with a base wood—typically alder, oak, or maple—and a flavor wood. The ratio of base wood to flavor wood tends to be between 50 to 70 percent base wood to 30 to 50 percent flavor wood. Pellets are blended in this fashion to ensure that they run through your grill properly. If the pellets are not blended correctly, they can create unsafe amounts of ash and even damage your grill.

Always be sure to use high-quality pellets. As the market grows, more and more types of pellets are being developed, and, without an industry standard, some of these are of poor quality and shouldn't be used. Many pellet grill companies make their own pellets, and you can usually feel comfortable using those. Grill manufacturers make their pellets with their grill in mind, and the pellets are tested during research and development. These are made to work specifically in your grill.

WOOD PELLET GRILLS AND SMOKE FLAVOR

The smoke flavor from a pellet grill is going to be different from what you are used to with a charcoal grill or wood smoker. Because of the complete burn that you perform with a pellet grill, the smoke is far lighter and slightly less potent. Most charcoal and wood smokers are not fan aided and depend on ambient air for their oxygen. These types of smokers give a heavier, creosote-tasting smoke.

Though pellet grills have a different flavor of smoke, that does not make it any less satisfying. There is no lack of smoke flavor on long-smoked cooks done on a pellet grill, but there's also no risk of creating an overpowering smoky flavor. Smoke flavor is also decreased when pellet grills move into higher temperatures, so for that family member who just doesn't like food too smoky, just cook hotter.

To get the optimal amount of smoke flavor from your grill, smoke at low temperatures for longer amounts of time. For those cooks where you really want to punch in the smoke, use a smoke tube from start to finish.

How Much Do You Need?

The amount of pellets you need is dependent on grill size and type, but generally you can expect to use about two pounds per hour on the smoke setting and up to five pounds per hour at a temperature of 500 degrees. Though it may seem like you are going to chew through pellets at high temperatures, it is actually quite the opposite. Low-and-slow cooks tend to use far more pellets than a quick, hot cook.

I advise you, no matter how long you plan to cook, to keep your hopper full. If needed, you can empty the hopper later, but this will ensure there is never a chance of running out of pellets and extinguishing the fire.

Proper Storage

How you store pellets is important. As I previously mentioned, hardwood pellets are held together by pressure alone, and moisture will wreak havoc on them. Always store your pellets indoors or in an airtight container. Many companies have pellet caddies available for storing your pellets, but you can always just head down to a hardware store and pick up a five-gallon bucket.

Along with your stored pellets, make sure to take care of the pellets in your hopper. Always cover your grill when not in use, and if you don't plan to use it for more than a few weeks, dump the hopper and run all pellets out of the auger.

TYPES OF WOOD

Use this handy chart when deciding which types of wood to use for the food you plan to cook on your grill.

WOOD	FLAVOR/AROMA	PAIRS WELL WITH
HICKORY	Heavy smoke, woodsy	All meats, nuts, fish, cheese, vegetables
MESQUITE	Heavy smoke, creosote	Beef, poultry, fish, cheese, game
ALDER	Subtle smoke, sweet	Beef, poultry, fish, baked goods, vegetables, game
MAPLE	Mild smoke	Pork, poultry, fish, baked goods, vegetables, game
OAK	Light smoke	Beef, fish, game
APPLE	Light smoke, sweet	Beef, pork, poultry, baked goods, vegetables
PECAN	Light smoke, nutty	Beef, pork, poultry, baked goods, vegetables
CHARCOAL	Smoky, charcoal	Beef, poultry, vegetables, game
COMPETITION BLENDS	Smoky, sweet	Everything
WALNUT	Smoky, earthy	Beef, lamb, vegetables
CHERRY	Light smoke, sweet	Pork, poultry, baked goods, vegetables

USING YOUR GRILL FOR THE FIRST TIME

Using your grill for the first time not only sets it up but also seasons the inside, removing any chemicals left over from manufacturing that might be lingering in the grill. Along with this, it gives you a firsthand opportunity to see how the grill runs. You are able to see how the grill first smokes heavily in startup, until ignition, before the temperature steadily rises. I recommend checking out your grill manufacturer's instructions for your first grill use, but most grills are very similar and have the same goal in mind: to fill your auger with pellets and deliver them to the firepot for ignition.

To start, you are going to want to fill your hopper with pellets. I always recommend a full hopper, no matter the cook time. Next, pull all items out of the inside of the grill, including the grates and drain pan, so you can see the firepot. Set the grill directly to high. This will turn the auger more frequently, allowing pellets to flow through the auger. Once you see pellets starting to drop into the firepot, turn the grill off. Now that the auger is fully primed, place all items back into the grill. Leave the grill lid open, turn the grill on, and set it to its lowest setting. You will see the grill begin to produce a heavy, white smoke after a short time. Within about four minutes, the smoke will dissipate, and you will hear the grill roar, indicating that the fire has been lit.

Once the fire has been established, close the grill lid and set your grill to a temperature above 350 degrees. Leave your grill at this set temperature for at least 30 minutes. This is the seasoning process. After those 30 minutes, your grill is ready to use. You can raise or lower the temperature to get the grill rolling right away, or shut it down and wait to get cooking.

LOW AND SLOW, HOT AND FAST, AND EVERYTHING IN BETWEEN

My favorite aspect of the pellet grill is by far the versatility. The pellet grill has a huge temperature range that gives you the ability to use many different cooking methods and styles. Though many people think of huge cuts of meat being smoked low and slow when we think of barbecue, this is by no means the only way to get great-tasting food. With the pellet grill, you can cook long and low, short and hot, right in the middle, or use a combination of all.

Different types of cooks will definitely give you some different results. From flavor to texture to tenderness, the way you cook will impact the way your final product comes out. Throughout the following section, I am going to briefly touch on some easy cooks that will put you on your way. This table gives you a brief estimated time and temperature for different cuts of meat—even multiple options for the same one. This is intended to give you a base of recipes that can be used at any time, not just when you want to create an extravagant meal. Prep these meats with your favorite rub, or one of those found in chapter 6, and go! Many of the rubs and sauces in chapter 6 are used in recipes throughout this book—feel free to use as much or as little of them as you like. Yield amounts for rubs and sauces are given at the beginning of each recipe.

YOUR GUIDE TO SMOKING

FOOD	SMOKER TEMP	SMOKE TIME	INTERNAL TEMP
Chicken			
BONELESS & SKINLESS BREAST	350°F	25 to 30 minutes	170°F
BONE-IN BREAST	350°F	45 minutes	170°F
BONE-IN THIGHS, DRUMSTICKS	350°F 275°F	45 minutes 1 hour 30 minutes to 2 hours	170°F
CHICKEN WINGS	375°F	20 minutes	170°F
WHOLE	375°F	1 hour 20 minutes	170°F
Turkey			
BREASTS	325°F	50 minutes	170°F
DRUMSTICKS	325°F	40 minutes	170°F
SPATCHCOCKED	350°F	2 hours	170°F
WHOLE	375°F	1 hour 30 minutes to 2 hours	170°F

FOOD	SMOKER TEMP	SMOKE TIME	INTERNAL TEMP
Beef			
2" STEAK, RARE	500°F	10 minutes per side	135°F
2" STEAK, MEDIUM	500°F	12 minutes per side	145°F
2" STEAK, WELL	500°F	15 minutes per side	155°F
BRISKET	225°F	14 to 18 hours	190°F
TRI-TIP, MEDIUM	375°F	45 minutes	145°F
Lamb			
LAMB CHOPS	350°F	25 minutes	145°F
Pork			
BABY BACK RIBS	225°F / 275°F	5 to 6 hours / 3 to 4 hours	200°F
PORK CHOPS	375°F / 275°F	10 minutes per side / 45 minutes	145°F
PORK TENDERLOIN	180°F	2 to 4 hours	145°F
PULLED PORK	225°F	16 to 18 hours	203°F
Seafood			
16- TO 32-OUNCE SALMON FILLET	325°F / 180°F	25 minutes / 4 hours	145°F
CATFISH FILLET	300°F	25 minutes	145°F
LOBSTER TAILS	400°F	20 minutes	145°F
OYSTERS IN THE SHELL	375°F	10 to 20 minutes	N/A
TUNA STEAKS	500°F	3 minutes per side	N/A
Produce			
GRILLED ASPARAGUS	325°F	10 minutes	N/A
PEACHES	375°F	7 minutes	N/A
POTATO WEDGES	375°F	45 minutes	N/A

KEEPING YOUR PELLET GRILL IN TIP-TOP CONDITION

Caring for your grill is important to protect your investment for years to come, but it's also necessary for proper performance. This section covers how to take care of your grill from the moment you shut it down, including how it should be stored.

Turning Off the Grill

Turning off the grill is about as basic as it seems. Shut your grill off when cooking is complete. Leave the lid shut and let it go. Many of today's pellet grills come standard with a shutdown cycle, so do not be surprised when the fan keeps running even after you turn the grill off.

If you do not foresee yourself using the grill again in the next couple of weeks, dump the hopper and run out the remaining pellets in the auger. Many newer grills have a hopper dump feature included, but if yours doesn't, an old plastic cup works great.

Cleaning the Firepot

There are a few ways to clean your grill's firepot, but what is important is that you *do* clean the firepot. The functionality of your grill is heavily influenced by airflow. Swings in temperature, low temperatures, high temperatures, and everything in between can be affected by a dirty firepot. Too much ash can block holes and significantly decrease the amount of air getting to the firepot.

Some of the newest grills on the market have simple ash cleanouts or dumps. There are some that work better than others, but it is a definite time-saver. For grills without a cleanout, there are a couple of options. The first is to vacuum the grill out with a Shop-Vac when cool. The second option is a little dirtier, but it gets the job done. Using a spoon, you can simply scoop out any ash from the firepot.

Cleaning the Grill Grates

The first rule of cleaning your grill grates is no steel brushes. Though steel brushes are cheap and easy to find, they can damage your grill—not to mention the horror stories of bristles getting lodged in people's throats when they eat food that was cooked on a steel brush–cleaned grill.

The easiest and safest way to clean your grates is at high heat with a damp rag. Use tongs or something else to hold the rag and rub it across the grates. Another easy hack is to ball up some aluminum foil and rub it across the grates.

For those of you looking for a brush-type tool, look for wooden grate scrapers or a palmyra brush that has bristles that are safe and clean.

Cleaning the Drain Pan

How you clean your drain pan depends on the style of the pan. One thing that applies no matter what is that your pan needs to be cleaned after about every 40 pounds of pellets or after a really greasy cook.

The easiest and most universal way to clean your pan is with a scraper. A paint scraper actually works great. Scrape all that gunk into the trash can and forget about it. For those of you with a traditional drain pan without plates, cover your pan with foil for easy cleanup. Do not cover your pan if you have a direct-flame option on your grill.

Storing the Grill

After your grill has cooled, you will want to protect it before storing it. This can be as simple as placing a cover over your grill. Some people pull their grills into a garage or shed when not in use. If you ever bring your grill indoors, make sure the fire is completely out first.

THE RECIPES

The next few chapters are the meat and potatoes of this book, pun intended. The following recipes were created with *you* in mind. These recipes are both simple and delicious. I have compiled them with the goals of limited prep time and limited effort in mind. The recipes in this book may be ones that you use for your next Super Bowl party, but are just as easily used for a weeknight dinner.

When I say "easy," I'm talking about the process. Easy recipes are often some of the most flavorful ones and give you a launching point for your own creations. These recipes will give you the skill set for truly mastering your pellet grill.

All the recipes in this book can be prepped in under 15 minutes. I know you don't want to toil away in the kitchen after a long day of work, and these recipes take that into account. In fact, most of the prep can be done during your grill's startup. So, set your grill to smoke, prep your food, and throw it on the grill.

In these recipes you will work with a limited ingredient list—fewer than

10 ingredients per recipe—to be able to get you moving in a hurry. Remember, you are going to let the grill do the work. Minimal ingredients allow the wood-fired smoke to penetrate the meats and give us an amazing result. On top of that, I will provide some super-easy recipes with five or fewer ingredients.

Every ingredient you will be using in this book is something you can easily find in your local market, focusing on common cuts and ingredients to give you the ultimate grilling experience.

Along with the recipes in this book, chapter 6 is all about rubs, seasonings, marinades, and sauces that will give you a base for all of your cooks—not only for these recipes, but for your own creations. Let's get started!

Texas Tri-Tip

P.22

BEEF, PORK, & LAMB

BASIC BRISKET

A great brisket is what many of us strive for when we begin smoking on our pellet grill. This tasty cut of meat is amazing when done right. I have spent hours working on my brisket game, using all sorts of techniques, and this is a tried-and-true method to create, with ease, the best brisket you will ever have.

Brisket comes in a couple of different cuts: the flat, the point, or the full packer, which contains both the flat and point. When using the full packer brisket, it is essential to trim much of the fat, especially the hard piece that runs between the point and flat.

In this recipe, you will be using a Texas Crutch. The Texas Crutch is a method of wrapping your meat to aid in the cook. This method keeps in moisture and allows you to cook at higher temperatures.

Prep time: **15 MINUTES**	Smoke time: **8 TO 12 HOURS** (plus 1 to 2 hours to rest)	Smoke temperature: **275°F**	Wood pellet flavor: **MESQUITE**

1 (12-pound) full packer brisket

2 tablespoons yellow mustard

Kosher salt

Freshly ground black pepper

1. Supply your smoker with wood pellets and follow the manufacturer's specific start-up procedure. Preheat the grill, with the lid closed, to 275°F.

2. Using a boning knife, remove all but about ½ inch of the large layer of fat that covers one side of the brisket. On the opposite side, remove the deckle, the hard piece of fat that separates the point from the flat part of the brisket.

3. Rub the brisket with the mustard, then sprinkle with a generous amount of salt and pepper and massage it into the meat.

4. Place the brisket directly on the grill grate, close the lid, and smoke for 6 to 10 hours, or until the internal temperature reaches 165°F.

5. Pull the brisket from the grill and wrap in either foil or butcher paper.

6. Return the wrapped brisket to the grill and cook for about 2 hours, or until the internal temperature reaches 190°F.

7. Remove the brisket from the grill and let rest for 1 to 2 hours, wrapped.

8. Unwrap the brisket. Using a slicing knife, separate the point from the flat part of the brisket and slice the flat part to serve.

Cooking tip: Speed up the process by turning your grill to a higher temperature—350°F works great, but only once the brisket is wrapped. Cooking an unwrapped brisket this hot will produce a great-tasting piece of leather. A quality slicing knife is a must-have for any kitchen. From brisket, to tenderloins, to turkey, the slicing knife is huge for those large meats. I use a Victorinox Fibrox for my slicer and all of my other knives.

TEXAS TRI-TIP

Texas is not known for tri-tip, but for this recipe, you will be using the Texas Crutch method again (see page 20). You want to hold those juices in after pumping the cut full of smoke flavor.

Tri-tip is my favorite cut of beef. It is primarily found on the West Coast, but these days, anything is available on the Internet. Omaha Steaks is a great option, along with many more.

Prep time: **10 MINUTES**	Smoke time: **3 HOURS** (plus 10 to 15 minutes to rest)	Smoke temperature: **180°F AND 375°F**	Wood pellet flavor: **HICKORY**

1 (1½-pound) tri-tip roast

Rosemary-Garlic Seasoning (page 85)

½ cup apple juice

Cooking tip: This is a perfect cook to use your smoke tube. Light the tube full of pellets right before you begin cooking. Throw the tube on when you put on the tri-tip and let that smoke soak in.

1. Supply your smoker with wood pellets and follow the manufacturer's specific start-up procedure. Preheat the grill, with the lid closed, to 180°F.

2. Rub the roast with a generous amount of the seasoning, massaging it into the meat, and set directly on the grill grate.

3. Close the lid and smoke for 2 to 2½ hours, or until the internal temperature reaches 115°F. Pull the tri-tip from the grill and place on a large piece of aluminum foil or butcher paper. Pour the apple juice over top and wrap tightly.

4. Increase the grill temperature to 375°F and return the tri-tip to the grill. Smoke for about 30 minutes, or until the internal temperature reaches 140°F.

5. Remove the tri-tip from the grill and let rest for 10 to 15 minutes before unwrapping, slicing, and serving.

SEARED NEW YORK STRIP

Serves 4

We all have our own favorite type of steak. New York Strip happens to be mine. When cooking dinner for myself, New York Strips are a usual suspect on the menu. With the perfect wood-fired sear, pair with potatoes or veggies and you have yourself a meal.

Prep time: **5 MINUTES**	Smoke time: **15 TO 20 MINUTES** (plus 5 minutes to rest)	Smoke temperature: **400°F**	Wood pellet flavor: **COMPETITION BLEND**

4 (1-inch-thick) New York Strip steaks

Beef and Brisket Rub (page 82)

1. Supply your smoker with wood pellets and follow the manufacturer's specific start-up procedure. Preheat the grill, with the lid closed, to 400°F.

2. Generously season the steaks with the rub, massaging it into the meat.

3. Place the steaks on the grill grate, close the lid, and cook for 7 to 10 minutes on one side. Flip the steaks and cook for another 7 to 10 minutes, or until their internal temperature reaches 145°F for medium-rare.

4. Remove the steaks from the grill and let rest for 5 minutes before serving.

Cooking tip: If your grill has an open-flame option, like a Pit Boss or Weber, this is the place to use it. The cook is the same, but the time will be reduced significantly. Place your New York Strips over the flame and sear them to temperature. This is the way to get those charred steaks you're used to getting from your gas or charcoal grill.

REVERSE-SEARED SIRLOIN

Serves 2 to 3

Reverse searing was something that I first heard of when I was the customer service manager at Traeger, but never did until years later. The reverse sear is a method where you first smoke your meat before giving it a nice, hot sear, sealing in all those juices.

In this recipe, you will be using sirloin steaks, which are often the most available and affordable at your local market. I love their flavor, and my family likes the fact that they are leaner than other cuts.

Prep time:	Smoke time:	Smoke temperature:	Wood pellet flavor:
10 MINUTES	**1 HOUR**	**180°F AND 400°F**	**HICKORY**

2 (6-ounce) sirloin steaks

Beef and Brisket Rub (page 82)

2 tablespoons butter

Cooking tip: Use this recipe for your favorite steaks. Like with other cooks, temperature is far more important than time in this one. Use the same temperature guidelines, and you're set to reverse sear a ribeye or tri-tip steak.

1. Supply your smoker with wood pellets and follow the manufacturer's specific start-up procedure. Preheat the grill, with the lid closed, to 180°F.

2. Generously season the steaks with the rub, massaging it into the meat.

3. Place the steaks on the grill grate, close the lid, and cook for about 50 minutes, or until the internal temperature reaches 125°F. Flip hallway through cooking. Remove the steaks from the grill and set aside.

4. Place a cast-iron skillet on the grill grate and increase the temperature to 400°F. Melt the butter in the skillet, add the steaks, and sear on all sides, using tongs to flip the steaks, for 5 to 10 minutes, or until the internal temperature reaches 145°F.

5. Remove the steaks from the skillet, slice, and serve immediately.

PELLET GRILL BEEF JERKY

Serves 6 to 8

If you have not had jerky from a pellet grill, you need it in your life. The flavor and texture are great, and you can make a whole batch of jerky for pellets on the dollar, compared to store brands. The best thing about pellet grill jerky is that it can be extremely easy. The part of this recipe that will take the longest is cutting the roast, so ask your butcher if they will do it for you.

Prep time: **15 MINUTES**	Smoke time: **4 TO 5 HOURS**	Smoke temperature: **180°F**	Wood pellet flavor: **MESQUITE**

1 pound top round roast

Kosher salt

Freshly ground black pepper

Cooking tip: Use whatever roast you like for this recipe. I use top round but am always up for something different. Oftentimes I simply go for the cheapest cut. I let the grill do the work and penetrate the meat with all that wood smoke.

1. Supply your smoker with wood pellets and follow the manufacturer's specific start-up procedure. Preheat the grill, with the lid closed, to 180°F. Light your smoke tube, if you have one, and place it in the grill.

2. Slice the roast against the grain into ¼-inch-thick pieces.

3. Lightly salt and pepper both sides of each slice.

4. Place the pieces directly on the grill grate. You may need to use more than one rack to fit them.

5. Close the lid and smoke the jerky for 4 to 5 hours, or until it is dry, but still bendable.

6. Remove and serve immediately. The jerky can be stored in an airtight container in the refrigerator for 2 to 3 weeks.

BEGINNER BURGERS

Serves 4

Burgers are another extremely simple cook. Mix the burgers the way you would if you were to cook them any other way. You can also sub in your favorite store-bought burgers if you want to speed things up even more. Grab some slices of cheese and some bacon and throw them on a couple of minutes before pulling the burgers off the grill for a killer bacon cheeseburger.

Prep time: **15 MINUTES**	Smoke time: **20 MINUTES**	Smoke temperature: **400°F**	Wood pellet flavor: **COMPETITION BLEND**

1 pound ground beef

1 egg

Beef and Brisket Rub (page 82)

Cooking tip: This is another cook that I prefer to do over an open flame. I had eaten burgers off the pellet grill my entire life and they never hit right until I opened up a flame broiler and gave them that char. Just keep an eye on them and cut a couple of minutes off your cook time and you will have a solid, flame-kissed burger.

1. Supply your smoker with wood pellets and follow the manufacturer's specific start-up procedure. Preheat the grill, with the lid closed, to 400°F.

2. In a medium bowl, combine the ground beef and egg, mixing thoroughly.

3. Divide the mixture into 4 individual patties and season both sides with the rub to taste.

4. Place the burgers on the grill grate, close the lid, and cook for 10 minutes, then flip and continue to cook for another 10 minutes, or until the internal temperature reaches 145°F.

5. Serve immediately on a bun with any of your favorite burger toppings.

PELLET PULLED PORK

Good pulled pork is awesome and easy. I love the effortlessness with which I can rub the pork, throw it on the grill, and wait. The key to great pulled pork is patience. This is a long, low-and-slow cook. If you try to speed it up, you risk not being able to pull the meat.

Prep time: **10 MINUTES**	Smoke time: **12 TO 16 HOURS** (plus 1 hour to rest)	Smoke temperature: **250°F**	Wood pellet flavor: **HICKORY**

1 (6- to 8-pound) bone-in pork shoulder

2 tablespoons honey mustard

Sweet Brown Sugar Rub (page 88)

Cooking tip: This recipe is written with sweet uses in mind, like sandwiches and sliders. If you are looking to change up the flavor for things like tacos and eggs, swap the honey mustard for yellow mustard and the Sweet Brown Sugar Rub for Poultry Rub (page 84). The mustard has minimal effect on taste, but a sweet or spicy mustard comes through.

1. Supply your smoker with wood pellets and follow the manufacturer's specific start-up procedure. Preheat the grill, with the lid closed, to 250°F.

2. Rub the pork shoulder with the mustard and season with a generous amount of the rub, massaging it into the meat.

3. Place the pork shoulder on the grill grate, close the lid, and smoke for 12 to 16 hours, or until the internal temperature reaches 203°F.

4. Remove the shoulder from the grill and let rest for 1 hour or more, until you're able to pull the pork with your hands without burning yourself.

5. Pull out the bone and pull the pork apart, using just your fingers.

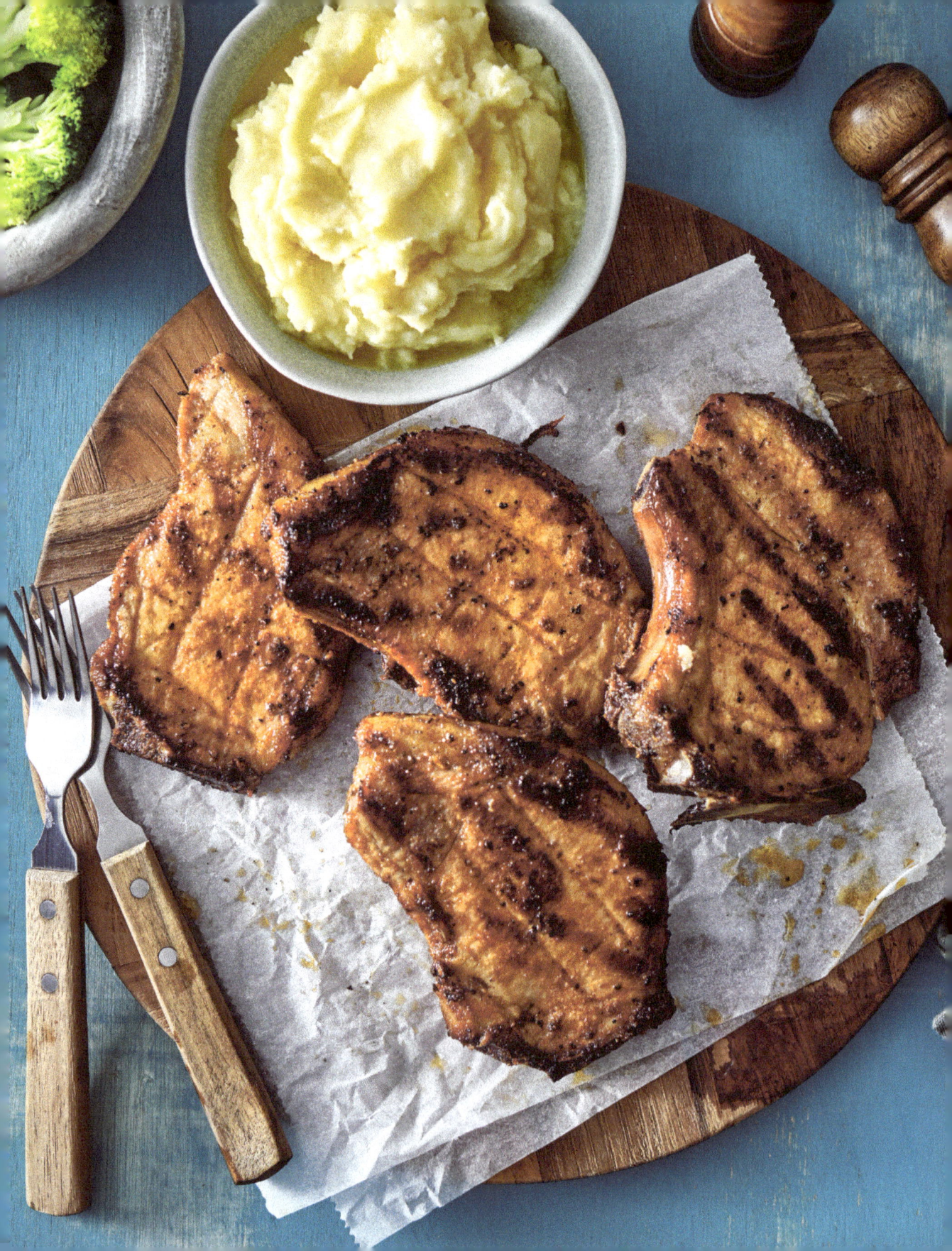

WOOD-FIRED PORK CHOPS

I don't cook pork chops as often as I should. This salty and flavorful cut is an easy cook as much as it is a tasty one. You can use your favorite cut, bone-in or boneless, or whatever is on sale. The prep is minimal, but the payoff is great. Serve the pork chops with mashed potatoes and broccoli, and you have yourself a simple weeknight meal.

Prep time: **5 MINUTES**	Smoke time: **35 MINUTES** (plus 5 minutes to rest)	Smoke temperature: **300°F**	Wood pellet flavor: **PECAN**

4½ pounds pork chops

Sweet Brown Sugar Rub (page 88)

1. Supply your smoker with wood pellets and follow the manufacturer's specific start-up procedure. Preheat the grill, with the lid closed, to 300°F.

2. Season the pork chops with the rub to taste.

3. Set the chops directly on the grill grate, close the lid, and cook for about 35 minutes, or until the internal temperature reaches 145°F. Flip the chops halfway through cooking.

4. Remove the pork chops from the grill and let rest for 5 minutes before serving.

Cooking tip: For a smoky pork chop, smoke the chops for about 1 hour before turning the temperature to 300°F. This will cut your cook time at 300°F by about 10 minutes and give you extra wood-fired flavor.

SMOKIN' HOT PORK TENDERLOINS

Serves 4 to 6

Tenderloins are a mainstay of pellet grilling. In their early efforts to sell the pellet grill, Joe and Randy Traeger and their team would use pork tenderloins, along with chicken, to give people the taste of safe and easy wood-fired barbecue.

I often cook tenderloins at home, and this is the way I like to do it. Smoking at 225°F will create tons of smoke flavor that won't take all night. With my family's busy extracurricular schedule, I can throw a tenderloin on the grill after work, and it is done at about the same time the whole family gets home.

Prep time: **5 MINUTES**	Smoke time: **2 TO 3 HOURS** (plus 10 minutes to rest)	Smoke temperature: **225°F**	Wood pellet flavor: **APPLE**

2 (1-pound) pork tenderloins

Spicy Rub (page 87)

Cooking tip: This is another cook that you can use your smoke tube for. Also, if you can, use a torch for lighting the smoke tube; that is my preferred option. I have spent far too much time with fluids and starters that rarely work and leave a smell.

1. Supply your smoker with wood pellets and follow the manufacturer's specific start-up procedure. Preheat the grill, with the lid closed, to 225°F.

2. Generously season the tenderloins with the rub, massaging it into the meat.

3. Place the tenderloins directly on the grill grate, close the lid, and smoke for 2 to 3 hours, or until the internal temperature reaches 145°F.

4. Remove the tenderloins from the grill and let rest for 10 minutes.

5. Slice the tenderloins and serve.

SWEET SMOKED HAM

There are a lot of ways to spice up a basic store-bought ham, and the best is on the pellet grill. This sweet ham recipe is guaranteed to be a hit at your next holiday party. Mixing the sweet flavor of maple with the salty, smoky flavor of the ham is always unbelievable. Though the ham you get at the store is likely presmoked, your pellet grill does an amazing job of adding the perfect amount of smoke flavor without drying it out.

Prep time: **10 MINUTES**	Smoke time: **4 TO 5 HOURS** (plus 5 to 10 minutes to rest)	Smoke temperature: **180°F**	Wood pellet flavor: **MAPLE**

1 (8- to 10-pound) precooked ham

Sweet Brown Sugar Rub (page 88)

3 tablespoons maple syrup

1. Supply your smoker with wood pellets and follow the manufacturer's specific start-up procedure. Preheat the grill, with the lid closed, to 180°F.

2. Generously season the ham with the rub, massaging the rub all over the ham.

3. Place the ham in a shallow pan. Set the pan on the grill grate and close the lid.

4. After 1 hour, drizzle the ham with the maple syrup.

5. Smoke the ham for 4 to 5 hours, or until the internal temperature reaches 145°F.

6. Remove the ham from the grill and let rest for 5 to 10 minutes.

7. Thinly slice the ham and serve.

Cooking tip: Make sure you are using precooked ham. Fresh ham, though amazing, is cooked differently.

PELLET GRILL BACON

One thing that surprises many new pellet grill owners is that you can cook your bacon on a pellet grill. Not only does it taste great on the grill, but it is also an awesome recipe to try for one of your first cooks on a new grill. This greasy cook will season the inside of your grill. And the great thing about it is that, even though the bacon is still greasy, it is contained inside your grill outdoors. Never worry about being burned by bacon grease again.

Smoke time:	Smoke temperature:	Wood pellet flavor:
20 MINUTES	**325°F**	**CHERRY**

1 pound thick-sliced pork bacon

1. Supply your smoker with wood pellets and follow the manufacturer's specific start-up procedure. Preheat the grill, with the lid closed, to 325°F.

2. Place the bacon slices directly on the grill grate. You will likely need multiple grates, and make sure the bacon does not go past the drain pan.

3. Close the lid and smoke the bacon for about 20 minutes, or until the bacon reaches your preferred doneness.

4. Serve immediately.

Cooking tip: Bacon racks are an awesome, but not essential, accessory. These racks give you room for plenty of bacon and catch the grease. One thing you will learn on your first bacon cook is how greasy it is and how easily the grease is contained.

LEG OF LAMB

Leg of lamb is a cut that I do not cook often, but when I do, it's a showstopper. The wood pellet smoke is the perfect complement to this cut. Lamb has a gamier taste than most of the popular meats that you see in the grocery store, so smokier woods like hickory and mesquite always pair well with lamb.

Prep time: **15 MINUTES**	Smoke time: **5 TO 7 HOURS** (plus 20 to 30 minutes to rest)	Smoke temperature: **180°F AND 400°F**	Wood pellet flavor: **MESQUITE**

1 (6- to 8-pound) boneless leg of lamb

2 tablespoons olive oil

Rosemary-Garlic Seasoning (page 85)

Cooking tip: The ultimate companion to lamb is mint jelly. Serve some on the side for a perfect dipping sauce.

1. Supply your smoker with wood pellets and follow the manufacturer's specific start-up procedure. Preheat the grill, with the lid closed, to 180°F.

2. Rub the lamb with the olive oil and then rub with a generous amount of the seasoning, rubbing underneath and around any netting.

3. Place the lamb directly on the grill grate and close the lid.

4. Smoke at 180°F for 4 to 6 hours, or until the internal temperature reaches 130°F.

5. Increase the temperature to 400°F and continue smoking for 45 minutes to 1 hour, or until the internal temperature reaches 145°F.

6. Remove the lamb from the grill and let rest for 20 to 30 minutes.

7. Remove any netting, slice, and serve.

LAMB KEBABS

Kebabs are a great way to make a meat cook into an entire meal. My wife often complains that all I worry about when cooking is the meat. This is true, but any chance I get to cook everything on the grill at once, I take it. Kebabs are one of my favorite ways to get it all done in one shot—and they cook quickly.

Prep time: **15 MINUTES**	Smoke time: **15 MINUTES**	Smoke temperature: **400°F**	Wood pellet flavor: **MESQUITE**

1 (2-pound) leg of lamb, cut into 1-inch cubes

½ white onion, cut into 1-inch pieces

1 green bell pepper, cut into 1-inch pieces

1 red bell pepper, cut into 1-inch pieces

½ pound cherry tomatoes

Kosher salt

Freshly ground black pepper

Cooking tip: Swap out the salt and pepper for your favorite rub. Of course, rosemary-based rubs are great with lamb, but so are beef and game rubs.

1. If using wooden skewers, soak them in water for 30 to 60 minutes.

2. Supply your smoker with wood pellets and follow the manufacturer's specific start-up procedure. Preheat the grill, with the lid closed, to 400°F.

3. Prepare the kebabs, making sure to leave 2 to 3 inches at either end: Thread the skewers alternating lamb, onion, lamb, green bell pepper, lamb, red bell pepper, lamb, cherry tomato, lamb, leaving a small gap between each ingredient.

4. Season the kebabs with salt and pepper to taste.

5. Place the kebabs on the grill grate, close the lid, and cook for about 15 minutes, or until the internal temperature of the meat reaches at least 140°F.

6. Remove the kebabs from the grill and serve immediately.

RACK OF LAMB

Roasted rack of lamb is a classic dish and one that is always a hit around Easter and Passover. Use this recipe for your perfect springtime meal. This roasted rack of lamb takes just a short time to prep and cook. All of this with the taste of wood fire, and you and your family are set!

Prep time: **10 MINUTES**	Smoke time: **1 HOUR** **30 MINUTES** (plus 20 to 30 minutes to rest)	Smoke temperature: **400°F**	Wood pellet flavor: **HICKORY**

1 (2-pound) rack of lamb

2 tablespoons olive oil

Rosemary-Garlic Seasoning (page 85)

Cooking tip: Lamb is one of the meats that I will cook almost exclusively on a pellet grill. There are some who cook it great other ways, but the pellet grill is a surefire way to have a solid meal, no matter what.

1. Supply your smoker with wood pellets and follow the manufacturer's specific start-up procedure. Preheat the grill, with the lid closed, to 400°F.

2. Score the fat portion of the rack of lamb at the bottom of the rib meat in a crosshatch pattern.

3. Rub the rack with the olive oil and a generous amount of the seasoning, massaging it into the scored fat.

4. Set the lamb directly on the grill grate, fat-side down. Close the lid and smoke at 400°F for 1½ hours, until the internal temperature reaches 145°F.

5. Remove the lamb from the grill and allow to rest for 20 to 30 minutes.

6. Slice and serve individual ribs.

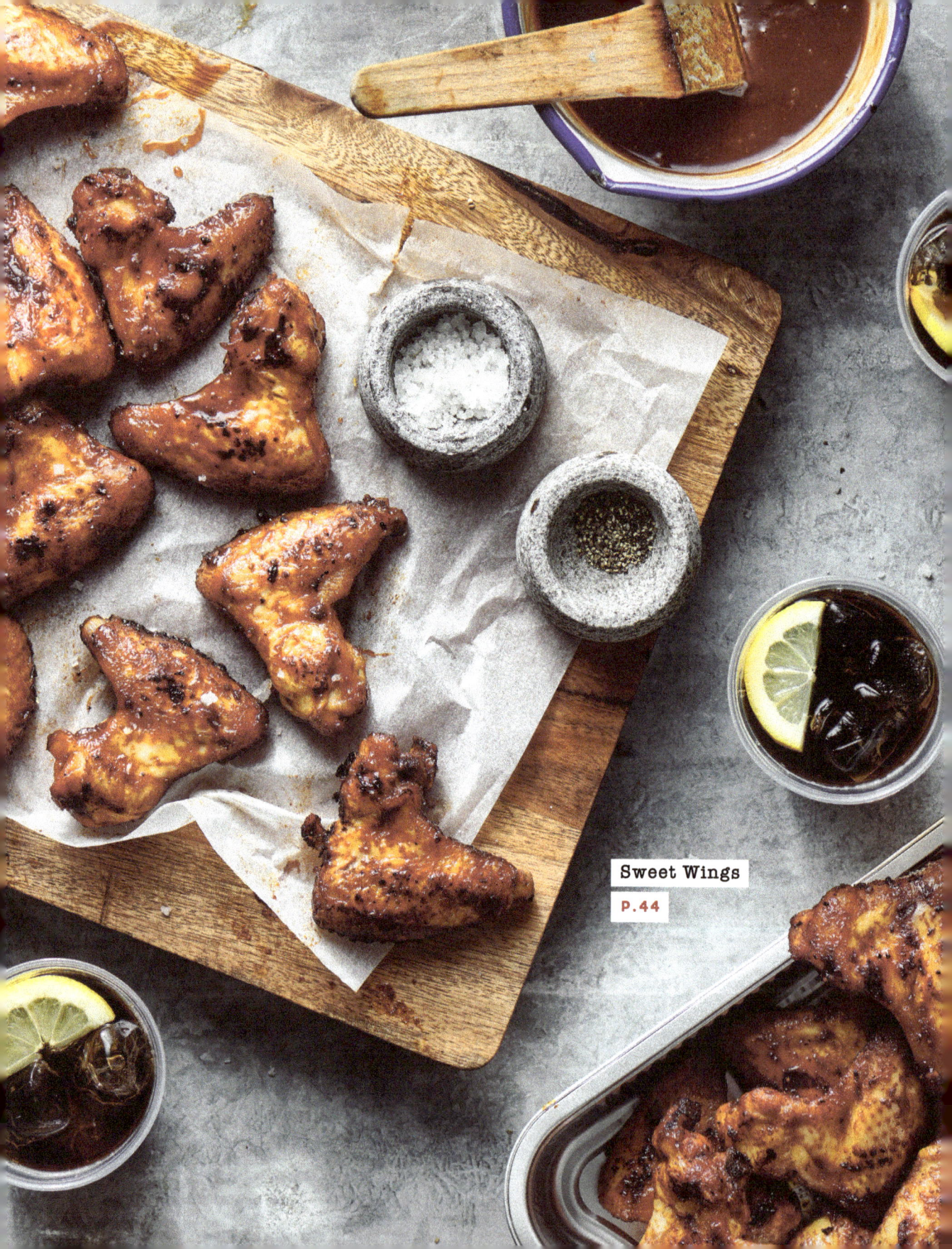

Sweet Wings
P.44

POULTRY

WHOLE CHICKEN

If you want a quick and basic cook that will feed your family and likely give you leftovers, this recipe for a whole chicken is it. Growing up, my family would have pellet-grilled chicken every week. I remember my mom prepping chicken when my dad was about to head home from work so dinner would be ready right around 5:00. This traditional pellet grill meal will be one that serves you for years.

Prep time:	Smoke time:	Smoke temperature:	Wood pellet flavor:
10 MINUTES	**1 HOUR 15 MINUTES**	**450°F**	**COMPETITION BLEND**

1 whole chicken

2 tablespoons olive oil

Poultry Rub (page 84)

1. Supply your smoker with wood pellets and follow the manufacturer's specific start-up procedure. Preheat the grill, with the lid closed, to 450°F.

2. Rub the chicken with the olive oil and generously season with the rub.

3. Place the chicken on the grill grate, close the lid, and cook for 1 hour 15 minutes, or until the internal temperature reaches 170°F in the thickest part of the breast.

4. Remove the chicken from the grill and carve for serving.

Cooking tip: Whole chicken is one of the greasier cooks you will do on your grill. Whole chickens, bacon, pulled pork, and brisket are ones I recommend you clean your drain pan after. Most cooks, especially small cuts, allow you to go multiple cooks without cleaning the pan, but anyone who has smoked out their neighbors with burning grease smoke knows how necessary cleaning the pan is.

GRILLED CHICKEN BREASTS

My family and I love chicken breasts. They are likely one of our most frequently cooked items. The flavor is great, and the convection of the pellet grill keeps the breasts moist. You can also do tons with a chicken breast. The ability to use different rubs and sauces allows you to pair breasts with just about any meal. This recipe is a basic one that can be expanded on. Just about all of the rubs in chapter 6 can be used on chicken, and so can many of the spices in your pantry.

Prep time: **5 MINUTES**	Smoke time: **25 MINUTES**	Smoke temperature: **350°F**	Wood pellet flavor: **HICKORY**

2½ pounds boneless, skinless chicken breasts

Poultry Rub (page 84)

1. Supply your smoker with wood pellets and follow the manufacturer's specific start-up procedure. Preheat the grill, with the lid closed, to 350°F.

2. Generously season the chicken with the rub.

3. Place the chicken on the grill grate, close the lid, and cook for about 25 minutes, or until the internal temperature reaches 170°F in the thickest part of the breast.

4. Remove the chicken from the grill and serve immediately.

Cooking tip: Take care not to overcook your boneless, skinless chicken breasts. This cut is one that can dry out easily if cooked too long. If you do find that you overcooked your chicken breasts, grab your favorite barbecue sauce and eat up.

SMOKED CHICKEN THIGHS

Serves 4

I am a total white-meat guy, but that does not mean that I can't get down with some dark meat every now and again, especially if it's at someone else's request. These little guys that look like pillows are an easy cook, and they go down just as easy. Chicken thighs are another one of those simple cooks that can give you and your crew a quick and tasty dinner.

To add some flavor to your thighs, throw on some barbecue sauce. My favorites are the Five Monkeys and Louisiana Grills lines of sauces. Five Monkeys has an Orange Chili that pairs amazingly with chicken dishes and is my absolute favorite.

Prep time: **5 MINUTES**	Smoke time: **1 HOUR 30 MINUTES** (plus 10 minutes to rest)	Smoke temperature: **180°F AND 375°F**	Wood pellet flavor: **OAK**

4 bone-in, skin-on chicken thighs

Kosher salt

Freshly ground black pepper

Cooking tip: One of my favorite things to do with poultry is to rub the seasoning under the skin. This can be done with most cuts, including thighs. Slowly work your fingers in between the skin and the meat. Once you have worked the skin away from the meat, rub the seasoning in the area between the two.

1. Supply your smoker with wood pellets and follow the manufacturer's specific start-up procedure. Preheat the grill, with the lid closed, to 180°F.

2. Season the chicken with salt and pepper to taste.

3. Place the chicken directly on the grill grate, close the lid, and smoke for 1 hour.

4. Set the grill to 375°F and continue cooking for about 30 minutes, or until the internal temperature of the thighs reaches 170°F.

5. Remove the chicken from the grill and let rest for 10 minutes before serving.

LEMON PEPPER CHICKEN BREAST

Texas Tri-Tip (page 22) and Bri & Chloe's Baby Shrimp (page 59) are my highlight reel, but I am so much more a Cal Ripken kind of guy. Chicken breast is the Iron Man cook. It's great tasting and healthy (and it tastes like chicken!).

There are so many ways to do a great chicken breast, but this is among my favorites. It is hot, fast, and full of flavor, and the colorful and crispy skin is always a crowd favorite. This recipe came straight from my teenage daughters and their friends' recommendations. With that kind of approval, you know it's good. This chicken is perfect with a green salad with vinaigrette on the side.

Prep time:	Smoke time:	Smoke temperature:	Wood pellet flavor:
10 MINUTES	**45 MINUTES**	**350°F**	**HICKORY**

3 pounds bone-in chicken breast

2 tablespoons olive oil

1 tablespoon lemon pepper

Kosher salt

Cooking tip: Rub your seasoning underneath the skin. It is very easy to work between the skin and the meat. This will work the flavor right into the meat.

1. Supply your smoker with wood pellets and follow the manufacturer's specific start-up procedure. Preheat the grill, with the lid closed, to 350°F.

2. Rub the chicken with the olive oil and season with the lemon pepper and salt to taste.

3. Place the chicken on the grill grate, close the lid, and cook for about 45 minutes, or until the internal temperature reaches 170°F in the thickest part of the breast.

4. Remove the chicken from the grill and carve for serving.

CHICKEN QUARTERS

If you want to make a full meal out of your protein, chicken quarters are for you. This was, and is, a cut that we use to show people how good the food cooked on a pellet grill is. Oregon summer evenings are not the same without chicken quarters, coleslaw, and corn on the cob. Grab a slice of Hermiston watermelon and a local IPA and you have yourself the traditional meal of a Pacific Northwest Pellet Griller.

Prep time: **10 MINUTES**	Smoke time: **1 HOUR** (plus 10 minutes to rest)	Smoke temperature: **300°F**	Wood pellet flavor: **CHARCOAL**

4 chicken quarters

2 tablespoons olive oil

Poultry Rub (page 84)

1. Supply your smoker with wood pellets and follow the manufacturer's specific start-up procedure. Preheat the grill, with the lid closed, to 300°F.

2. Rub the chicken with the olive oil and season generously with the rub.

3. Place the chicken directly on the grill grate, close the lid, and smoke for 1 hour, or until the internal temperature reaches 170°F.

4. Remove the chicken and let rest for 10 minutes before serving.

Cooking tip: I love to cook these up when I'm having a party and I need to feed a lot of people. The great thing about this recipe and a pellet grill is that it can easily be doubled or tripled to feed more people. The controller will control the grill's temperature, and you won't need to add a second of additional time.

HEAVY METAL DRUMSTICKS

Drumsticks are my favorite dark meat. I love being able to grab one and go to town. I spend a lot of time experimenting with flavors on drumsticks because they have such good flavor on their own and taste amazing with a variety of rubs and seasonings.

My favorite way to make drumsticks is spicy. Spicy flavors make the drumsticks almost like wings, but they take much less effort.

Prep time:	Smoke time:	Smoke temperature:	Wood pellet flavor:
10 MINUTES	**20 MINUTES**	**400°F**	**PECAN**

1 pound chicken drumsticks

2 tablespoons olive oil

Spicy Rub (page 87)

Cooking tip: I really enjoy a char on my drumsticks. The char reminds me of the chicken dinners that I would have from my uncle's charcoal grill growing up. I used to spend a lot of time at my cousins's house as a kid, playing cards and watching *Star Wars*. For a while, they didn't have a pellet grill and used a Weber Kettle. As a pellet grill kid, this was different and interesting to me. Today, I get that flavor on my pellet grill, without drying out the chicken.

1. Supply your smoker with wood pellets and follow the manufacturer's specific start-up procedure. Preheat the grill, with the lid closed, to 400°F.

2. Rub drumsticks with the olive oil and liberally season with the rub.

3. Place the drumsticks on the grill grate, close the lid, and cook for about 20 minutes, or until the internal temperature reaches 170°F.

4. Remove the drumsticks from the grill and serve immediately.

SWEET WINGS

Wings are another amazing, solid chicken piece that goes with tons of different flavors—just ask Buffalo Wild Wings. I have been a football season ticket holder at Oregon State University for some time, and Buffalo Wild Wings is a regular stop for my dad, brother, and me before games. Though I love the spicy flavors, my dad and brother love the sweet ones. I have grown an appreciation for these sweeter wings and have added them to my wing menu.

Prep time: **5 MINUTES**	Smoke time: **25 MINUTES**	Smoke temperature: **400°F**	Wood pellet flavor: **OAK**

1 pound split chicken wings

Sweet Brown Sugar Rub (page 88)

1 cup Honey BBQ Sauce (page 90)

3 tablespoons honey

Cooking tip: Mix your honey and barbecue sauce together and heat it in the microwave for about 25 seconds. This will make the liquid thinner and easier to spread over your wings. This is something you can do with all of your barbecue sauces when using them to baste or cover your meats. I love mixing in honey or maple syrup for extra flavor when making a sweet dish.

1. Supply your smoker with wood pellets and follow the manufacturer's specific start-up procedure. Preheat the grill, with the lid closed, to 400°F.

2. Season the wings with the sweet rub to taste and place the chicken on the grill grate.

3. Close the lid and cook for about 25 minutes, or until the internal temperature reaches 170°F.

4. Once cooked, move the wings to a large bowl. Cover with the barbecue sauce and honey and toss to coat the wings evenly with the sauce.

5. Serve immediately.

SIMPLE SMOKED TURKEY

Serves 10 to 14

Say it with me: "Turkey is not just for Thanksgiving." Turkey is one of my favorite things to make on the pellet grill. Every year, to this day, I look forward to my dad's Thanksgiving turkey, but I have to find a way to hold myself over during the rest of the year. Throughout the year I will try different methods of cooking my turkey. My days of managing customer service in the grilling industry made me obsessed with being able to tell my team the best way of cooking a turkey every November. Of them all, smoking is by far my favorite.

Prep time:	Smoke time:	Smoke temperature:	Wood pellet flavor:
10 MINUTES	**4 HOURS**	**180°F AND 350°F**	**HICKORY**

1 (13- to 16-pound) whole turkey

2 tablespoons olive oil

Poultry Rub (page 84)

Cooking tip: Use butter to baste your turkey during step 4. I leave a stick on my side shelf and hit the turkey about every 20 minutes or so. This not only will keep the turkey's skin from drying out and cracking but will give you more flavor than you can handle.

1. Supply your smoker with wood pellets and follow the manufacturer's specific start-up procedure. Preheat the grill, with the lid closed, to 180°F.

2. Coat the turkey with the olive oil and generously season with the rub. Rub the seasoning under the skin, if you can.

3. Place the turkey on the grill grate, close the lid, and smoke for 2½ hours.

4. Increase the temperature to 350°F and roast for about 1½ hours, or until the internal temperature reaches 170°F.

5. Remove the turkey from the grill and carve for serving.

ALL-AMERICAN ROAST TURKEY

If you want that traditional turkey but with a wood-fired twist, roast your turkey on your pellet grill. Even when you cook at higher temperatures, you will get that smoky taste. That wood-fired heat will surround and soak into your turkey any time it is on your grill.

This is the way to cook your turkey if you want it done fast, but still want to keep moisture and flavor. I have often been asked why we do not add a rotisserie to pellet grills to maintain even heat and keep the meat moist. The reason is because the grill does that on its own. Convection is what makes it happen and is what makes the pellet grill the best in the market.

Prep time: **15 MINUTES**	Smoke time: **2 HOURS 30 MINUTES** (plus 10 minutes to rest)	Smoke temperature: **375°F**	Wood pellet flavor: **OAK**

1 (13- to 16-pound) whole turkey

2 tablespoons olive oil

Poultry Rub (page 84)

Cooking tip: Make sure you check if your turkey is prebrined or not. Most popular brands like Butterball are prebrined, which I recommend for this recipe. If you have your own brine that you want to try with this recipe, make sure your bird isn't already brined.

1. Supply your smoker with wood pellets and follow the manufacturer's specific start-up procedure. Preheat the grill, with the lid closed, to 375°F.

2. Rub the turkey with the olive oil and generously season with the rub. Rub the seasoning under the skin, if you can.

3. Place the turkey directly on the grill grate, close the lid, and cook for 2½ hours, or until the internal temperature reaches 170°F.

4. Remove the turkey from the grill and let rest for 10 minutes.

5. Carve and serve.

TURKEY DRUMSTICKS

My family loves Disneyland, and one of my kids' favorite things to get while there are the giant turkey drumsticks. While this recipe is not the same as the park's, it definitely works to hold us over, every now and again.

There is something different about turkey legs. They are packed with all kinds of flavor on their own, and by adding that wood-smoke flavor from your pellet grill, you have a crowd-pleaser.

Prep time: **10 MINUTES**	Smoke time: **45 MINUTES**	Smoke temperature: **325°F**	Wood pellet flavor: **MESQUITE**

2 turkey drumsticks

2 tablespoons olive oil

Poultry Rub (page 84)

1. Supply your smoker with wood pellets and follow the manufacturer's specific start-up procedure. Preheat the grill, with the lid closed, to 325°F.

2. Rub the drumsticks with the olive oil and season with the rub to taste.

3. Place the drumsticks on the grill grate, close the lid, and cook for about 45 minutes, or until the internal temperature reaches 170°F.

4. Remove the drumsticks from the grill and serve immediately.

Cooking tip: You can also smoke your drumsticks at 180°F for an hour before turning your grill to 325°F. This will add to the amazing smoke flavor. Our goal is to ensure that the internal temperature reaches 170°, so adjust your cooking time accordingly.

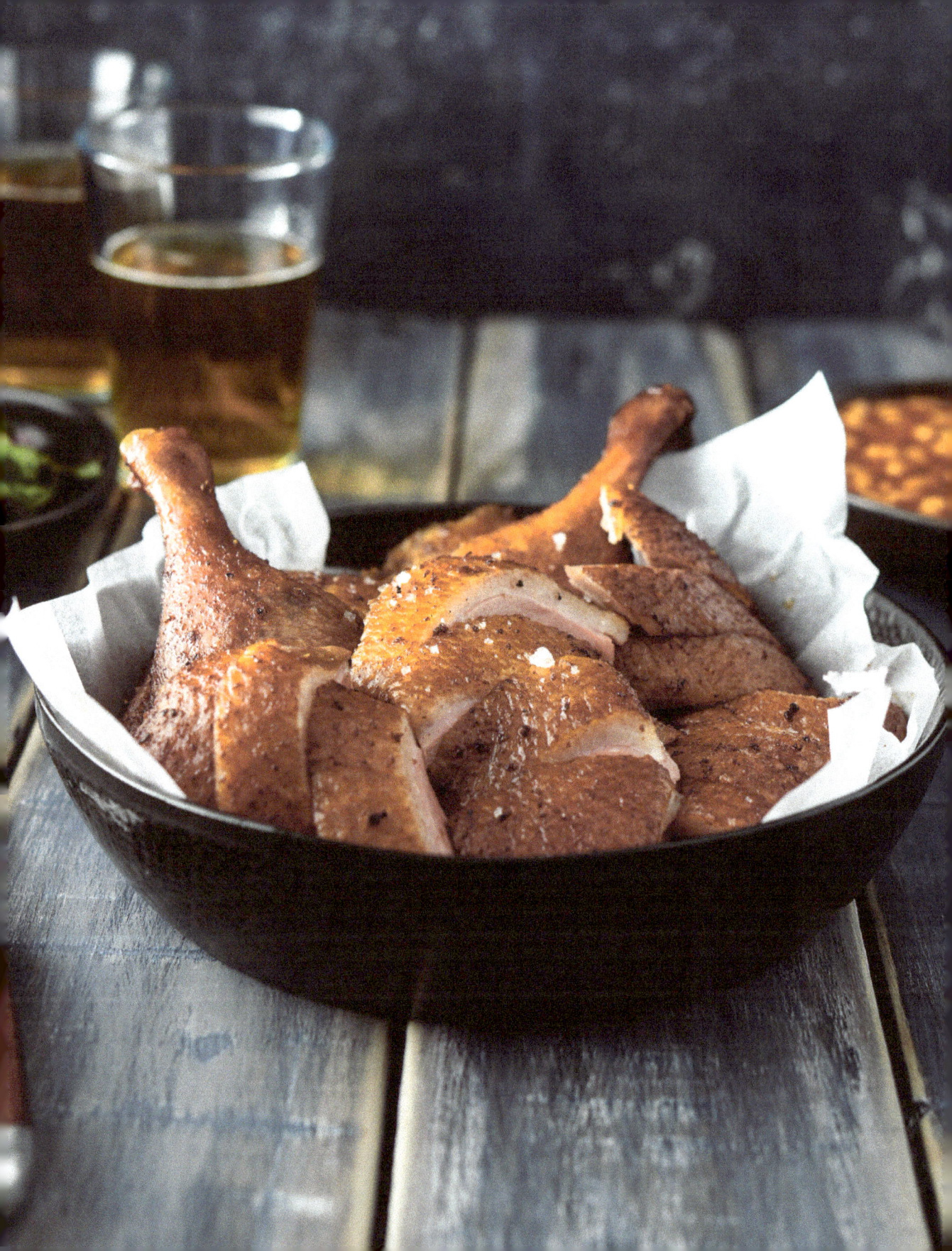

THE OREGON DUCK

I love to cook duck. Since my college days at Oregon State University, I have been known to cook one or two a year. The rival of my OSU Beavers is the University of Oregon Ducks. I always enjoy talking unfounded smack to my friends about the Ducks. My favorite way to poke fun is to cook a duck every year for the Oregon State football game. I serve it to Beavers and Ducks alike, and I always love to hear the compliments from the Ducks fans, right before the teams take the field.

Prep time:	Smoke time:	Smoke temperature:	Wood pellet flavor:
10 MINUTES	**1 HOUR 30 MINUTES**	**375°F**	**ALDER**

1 whole duck

2 tablespoons olive oil

Perfect Pork Rub (page 83)

1. Supply your smoker with wood pellets and follow the manufacturer's specific start-up procedure. Preheat the grill, with the lid closed, to 375°F.

2. Rub the duck all over with the olive oil and generously season with the rub, massaging it into the skin.

3. Place the duck on the grill, close the lid, and cook for 1½ hours, or until the internal temperature reaches 170°F in the thickest part of the breast.

4. Remove the duck from the grill and carve for serving.

Cooking tip: A large spatula or a fish spatula is a must-have for any committed griller. This accessory is my savior for whole poultry and large cuts of meat. The large spatula keeps your big cuts together and is much cleaner. No one wants meat and grease all over their porch.

SMOKED TURKEY BREAST

Serves 2 to 4

As I have mentioned before, I am a total white-meat guy. Whether it be chicken, turkey, or anything else, pass me a few good-size slices of the breast meat.

Smoked turkey breasts are a tasty cut and the perfect meal for a couple of people who love white meat. This recipe gives you a moist and flavorful turkey breast. The skin helps keep the moisture trapped, and the pellet grill's convection will do the rest.

Prep time:	Smoke time:	Smoke temperature:	Wood pellet flavor:
10 MINUTES	**1 HOUR 15 MINUTES**	**180°F AND 400°F**	**HICKORY**

1 (3-pound) skin-on turkey breast

2 tablespoons olive oil

Rosemary-Garlic Seasoning (page 85)

1. Supply your smoker with wood pellets and follow the manufacturer's specific start-up procedure. Preheat the grill, with the lid closed, to 180°F.

2. Rub the turkey breast with the olive oil and a generous amount of the seasoning.

3. Place the breast on the grill grate, close the lid, and smoke at 180°F for 1 hour.

4. Increase the grill temperature to 400°F and grill for about 15 minutes, or until the internal temperature reaches 170°F.

5. Remove the breast from the grill and serve immediately.

Cooking tip: I often use olive oil with my poultry. This helps keep the skin from cracking, but also works to crisp it. Oil on your poultry, at high temperatures, will help the skin tighten up and give you the crispy skin you are looking for.

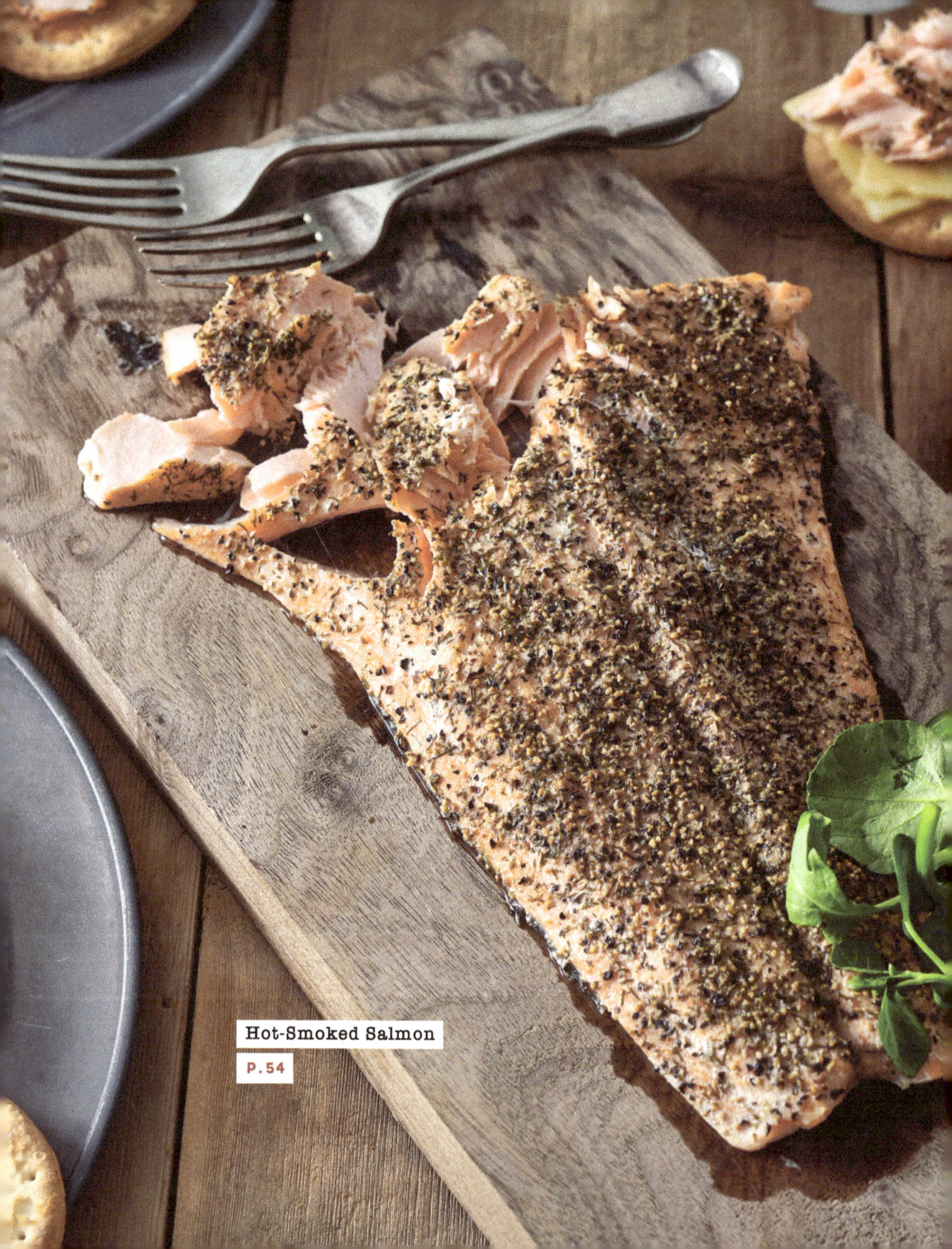

Hot-Smoked Salmon

P.54

SEAFOOD

HOT-SMOKED SALMON

There are two different methods of smoking, hot and cold. When using a pellet grill, you are hot smoking. This means that you are actually cooking while smoking, which allows you to have a quicker smoke, but also a fully cooked cut when pulling the food off the grill.

Hot-smoked salmon is amazing. I typically do some on my grill three to four times per year. It is one of my favorites and super easy. This version is served cold after refrigerating the cooked salmon overnight, but you can also serve it hot off the grill.

Prep time: **5 MINUTES**	Smoke time: **4 TO 5 HOURS** (plus overnight to chill)	Smoke temperature: **180°F**	Wood pellet flavor: **MESQUITE**

1 (1-pound) salmon fillet, skin-on

Superb Seafood Rub (page 86)

1. Supply your smoker with wood pellets and follow the manufacturer's specific start-up procedure. Preheat the grill, with the lid closed, to 180°F.

2. Sprinkle the salmon with the rub to taste.

3. Place the salmon on the grill grate, skin-side down. Close the lid and smoke for 4 to 5 hours, or until the salmon's internal temperature reaches 145°F.

4. Remove the salmon from the grill and let it cool. Tightly wrap it in plastic wrap, and refrigerate overnight before serving.

Cooking tip: There are tons of ways that you can serve your smoked salmon. My family's favorite is with butter crackers and slices of cheddar or Swiss cheese.

PEPE'S GRILLED SALMON

Salmon is my favorite fish. Fortunately for me, I grew up on it. Salmon is plentiful in the Pacific Northwest and it was a regular occurrence for my family to have salmon for dinner, especially on special occasions.

Currently, my son and I are the huge salmon fans in our house. Andrew Jr., or Pepe, as we refer to him, likes most of the meat I cook, but especially salmon. Recently, my local market started carrying Skuna Bay salmon. Oh, my gosh. While the girls will hold back a little, Pepe and I go all out on this moist and flavorful fish.

Prep time: **5 MINUTES**	Smoke time: **20 MINUTES**	Smoke temperature: **350°F**	Wood pellet flavor: **ALDER**

1 (2-pound) half salmon fillet, skin-on

Superb Seafood Rub (page 86)

1. Supply your smoker with wood pellets and follow the manufacturer's specific start-up procedure. Preheat the grill, with the lid closed, to 350°F.

2. Sprinkle the salmon with the rub to taste.

3. Place the salmon on the grill grate, skin-side down. Close the lid and grill for about 20 minutes, or until the internal temperature reaches 145°F.

4. Remove the salmon from the grill and serve immediately.

Cooking tip: Use a salmon spatula or an oversize spatula for salmon. A large spatula will prevent the fish from breaking as you pull it from the grill.

LOW-AND-SLOW SALMON

Salmon is far easier to make amazing than most people would guess. It takes on flavor well; you can work with your favorites to make dishes that you will be talking about for years. Marinating your salmon is a great way to do this. In this recipe, you will not only marinate but also cook at a low temperature, resulting in a moist, tasty fish.

I'm a busy guy, but I love cooking. With salmon being one of my favorite things to cook, I will cook it at a low temperature to give me time to pick up the kids from practice. Along with some frozen veggies, noodles, or rice, dinner is simple, and Mom and Dad are heroes.

Prep time: **5 MINUTES**	Smoke time: **50 MINUTES** (plus 20 minutes to marinate)	Smoke temperature: **260°F**	Wood pellet flavor: **ALDER**

1 (2-pound) half salmon fillet, skin-on

Carne Asada Marinade (page 89)

Sweet Brown Sugar Rub (page 88)

Cooking tip: It is easy to dry out your salmon, or any other fish, on any grill. I only cook my salmon by temperature. Flake tests are great for telling if your fish is done, but not necessarily done to the proper serving temperature.

1. Place the salmon and the marinade in a 1-gallon sealable bag or container of your choice. Marinate in the refrigerator for at least 20 minutes, and up to 24 hours.

2. Supply your smoker with wood pellets and follow the manufacturer's specific start-up procedure. Preheat the grill, with the lid closed, to 250°F.

3. Remove the salmon from the marinade. Discard the marinade. Pat dry the salmon with a paper towel and sprinkle generously with the rub.

4. Place the salmon on the grill grate, skin-side down. Close the lid and smoke for about 50 minutes, or until the internal temperature reaches 145°F.

5. Remove the salmon from the grill and serve immediately.

MICHAEL'S WOOD-FIRED SCALLOPS

Serves 4

I had never grilled scallops in my life until about 2018. I had just begun working for Pit Boss and Louisiana Grills and was getting heavily into grilling. I was always up for showing off my skills, learning new things, and teaching others.

My friend Michael was really into smoking at the time and currently cooks on a Pit Boss Austin XL. He lives in Ontario, Canada, and we frequently message back and forth about what we are cooking on our grills. The first time he visited me in Oregon, we grilled scallops. These were amazing on my Louisiana Grills LG700 and were done extremely fast.

Prep time: **10 MINUTES**	Smoke time: **10 MINUTES**	Smoke temperature: **375°F**	Wood pellet flavor: **MESQUITE**

1 pound large scallops

2 tablespoons olive oil

Superb Seafood Rub (page 86)

1. Supply your smoker with wood pellets and follow the manufacturer's specific start-up procedure. Preheat the grill, with the lid closed, to 375°F.

2. Coat the scallops with the olive oil and liberally season with the seafood rub.

3. Place the scallops directly on the grill grate, close the lid, and grill for 5 minutes per side.

4. Remove the scallops from the grill and serve immediately.

Cooking tip: Make sure you use large enough scallops for this recipe that they do not fall through the grill grate. If needed, run a wooden skewer through the scallops to prevent this.

BBQ TROUT

I don't fish much at all. My son and I have gone recently, but my skill has left me. Back in my twenties, I would fish with friends and drink beers. More often than not, we would pull trout out of the Abiqua Creek, just outside of town. We rarely took them home, but when big enough, it was a treat.

My parents love to fish and have brought back scores of trout, and it's from them that I learned and perfected cooking it. Mom and Dad would bring me and my two siblings home a good catch, and I would go about grilling or smoking mine.

Prep time: **5 MINUTES**	Smoke time: **25 MINUTES**	Smoke temperature: **325°F**	Wood pellet flavor: **HICKORY**

2 (1-pound) trout fillets, butterflied

Superb Seafood Rub (page 86)

1 lemon, sliced into rounds

1. Supply your smoker with wood pellets and follow the manufacturer's specific start-up procedure. Preheat the grill, with the lid closed, to 325°F.

2. Sprinkle the inside of the trout fillets with the seafood rub to taste.

3. Place the lemon slices inside the trout fillets.

4. Set the trout on the grill grate, close the lid, and grill for about 25 minutes, or until the internal temperature reaches 145°F.

5. Remove the trout from the grill and serve immediately.

Cooking tip: I typically rub my grill grates with oil prior to cooking fish. This helps to keep the skin from sticking to the grate, which can create a giant mess.

BRI & CHLOE'S BABY SHRIMP

Serves 4

When I was younger, I did not use my grill nearly as often as I do now. While my daughters, Brianna and Chloe, were young, I was doing most of my cooking indoors. I would use the stovetop to cook many of their dinners, especially while my wife was in school. This meal, however, was saved for when we could all have it together. Baby shrimp cooked in a lemon butter sauce was a favorite for our little family. The shrimp went great with pasta and frozen veggies.

When I started hammering down on the grill, I tried to find ways to cook everything outside. I soon turned this stovetop meal into a wood-fired, cast-iron recipe. Though the flavor is much the same, you do get some of the smoke flavor to come through. For more smoke flavor, set your grill to smoke for the last five or so minutes of cooking.

Prep time:	Smoke time:	Smoke temperature:	Wood pellet flavor:
10 MINUTES	**10 TO 15 MINUTES**	**400°F**	**OAK**

8 tablespoons (1 stick) butter

Juice of 1 lemon

Kosher salt

2 tablespoons dried dill weed

1 teaspoon garlic powder

1 pound baby shrimp

Cooking tip: Baby shrimp are usually precooked, and that is all I buy. This allows us to play with the flavor, but not have to cook them for too long.

1. Supply your smoker with wood pellets and follow the manufacturer's specific start-up procedure. Place a cast-iron skillet onto the grill and preheat, with the lid closed, to 400°F.

2. When the grill has reached temperature, melt the butter in the skillet.

3. Once the butter is melted, add the lemon juice, salt, dill weed, and garlic powder, and mix. Then add the shrimp.

4. Close the lid and braise the shrimp for 10 to 15 minutes, or until pink.

5. Remove the shrimp from the grill and serve immediately.

SPICY SHRIMP SKEWERS

Shrimp skewers are a definite crowd-pleaser. I love throwing a plate of these out at a party and watching them disappear. The best thing about these barbecue delights is that they are quite simple. The most time-consuming part of making these skewers is waiting on the wood skewers to soak. It is important to soak your skewers before using them on a grill, or those wood sticks might just catch fire.

Prep time: **10 MINUTES**	Smoke time: **10 MINUTES**	Smoke temperature: **400°F**	Wood pellet flavor: **HICKORY**

1 pound peeled and deveined shrimp, tails on

2 tablespoons olive oil

Spicy Rub (page 87)

1. Soak the skewers in water for 30 minutes.

2. Supply your smoker with wood pellets and follow the manufacturer's specific start-up procedure. Preheat the grill, with the lid closed, to 400°F.

3. Thread 4 to 5 shrimp per skewer.

4. Coat the shrimp with olive oil and season with the rub to taste.

5. Place the skewers on the grill grate, close the lid, and cook for about 5 minutes per side until the shrimp turn pink.

6. Remove the skewers from the grill and serve immediately.

Cooking tip: Make sure to use peeled shrimp. This will save you a ton of time plus eliminate the risk of a guest eating shrimp shells.

OYSTERS IN THE SHELL

Oysters are hit or miss for a lot of people. Myself, I love them. My favorite way to have them is cooked in the shell. They cook in their own juices and pack in the ocean flavor. Shuck the oysters to add whatever flavor you like. I like to prepare them with a little seafood rub and a lot of lemon.

Prep time: **10 MINUTES**	Smoke time: **10 TO 20 MINUTES**	Smoke temperature: **375°F**	Wood pellet flavor: **COMPETITION BLEND**

10 oysters, washed

Superb Seafood Rub (page 86)

Juice of 1 lemon

1. Supply your smoker with wood pellets and follow the manufacturer's specific start-up procedure. Preheat the grill, with the lid closed, to 375°F.

2. Set the oysters on the grill grate, close the lid, and cook for 10 to 20 minutes, until they open.

3. Remove the oysters from the grill and shuck them, disposing of the disconnected portion of the shell. Discard any oysters that didn't open.

4. Sprinkle the oysters liberally with the rub, and drizzle with the lemon juice. Serve immediately.

Cooking tip: I always use a butter knife and a leather glove to shuck my oysters. My dad uses an oyster knife, which is ideal to wedge into the shell, and it also usually has a nice wide handle perfect for the job.

GRILLED CRABS

In college, I worked for a local grocery store. (Roth's Fresh Market is known for quality local products and world-class service.) Every winter and early spring, Dungeness crab comes into season, and we would sell it like crazy.

I still go to Roth's at that time of year to pick up a few crabs. I make sure to ask for them to be cleaned, which saves me a lot of time, and I cook them on my pellet grill.

Prep time:	Smoke time:	Smoke temperature:	Wood pellet flavor:
5 MINUTES	**10 MINUTES**	**325°F**	**HICKORY**

2 Dungeness crabs, cleaned

8 tablespoons (1 stick) butter

Kosher salt

2 tablespoons dried dill weed

1 teaspoon garlic powder

1. Supply your smoker with wood pellets and follow the manufacturer's specific start-up procedure. Preheat the grill, with the lid closed, to 325°F.

2. Place the crabs on the grill grate, close the lid, and cook for about 10 minutes, or until the crab shell turns a reddish pink.

3. While the crabs are cooking, melt the butter in a microwave-safe bowl in the microwave or on the stovetop. Add the salt, dill weed, and garlic powder to the melted butter and mix.

4. Remove the crabs from the grill and serve with the seasoned butter.

Cooking tip: Baste your crab with butter while cooking. This will keep them from burning and drying out.

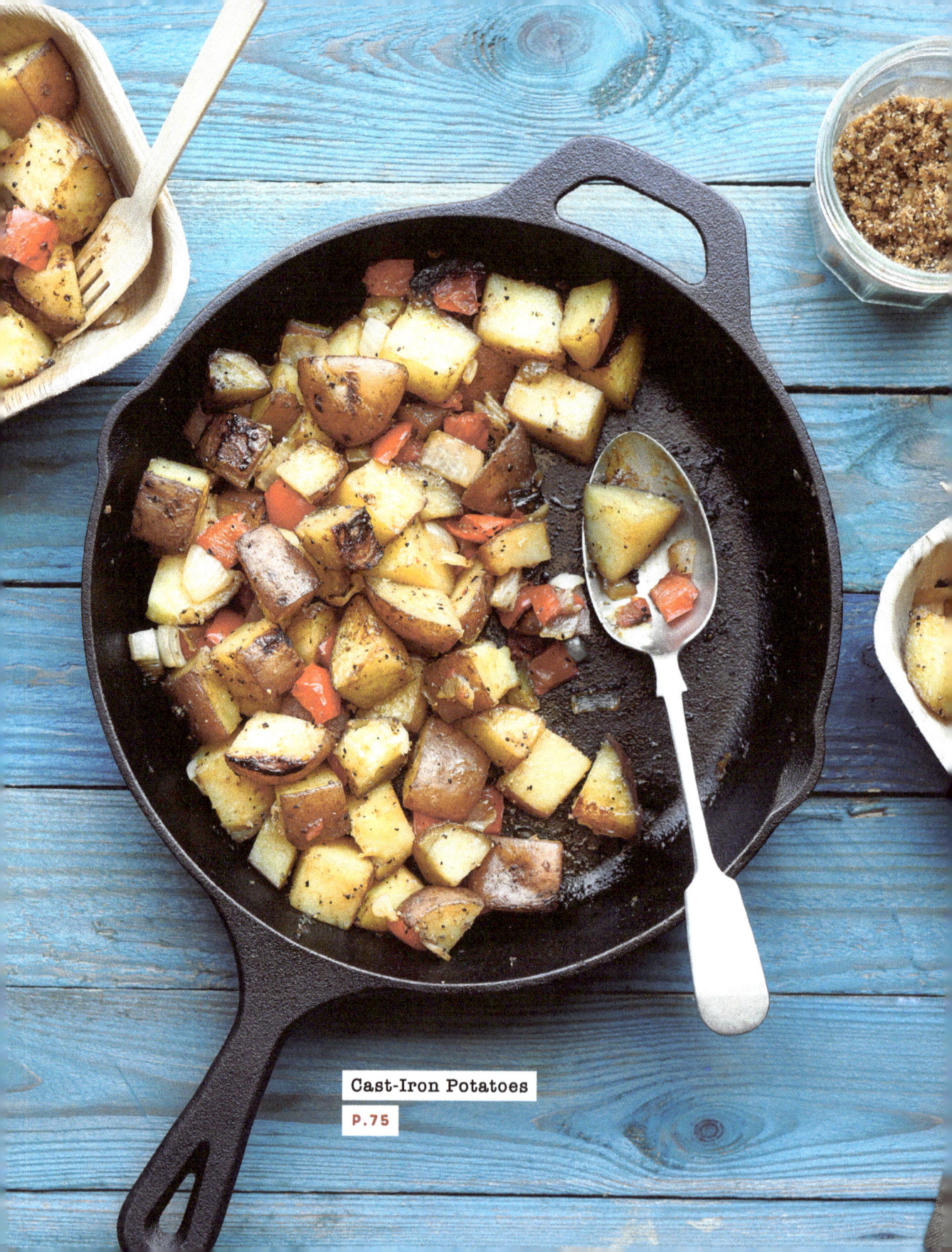

Cast-Iron Potatoes

P.75

SIDES

PNW CHILI

Your grill is able to do anything you can do inside on the stovetop. I rarely cook indoors because of the ability to cook an entire meal on the grill at once, meat and veggies included. This recipe is made even easier because it's cooked in one pot. Recipes that are known for the stovetop, like chili, are made easy and delicious on the grill.

In the Pacific Northwest, we have taken to a different style of barbecue. This style revolves around using wood fire to create culinary masterpieces that you would not typically find on a grill. Though not quite a culinary masterpiece, chili is something that we typically do inside, but in the PNW we grab a raincoat and head to the grill.

To make this recipe, you will use a store-bought chili mix packet. I usually use the store brand, but McCormick makes a solid mix as well. If you are a chili pro or once you have the process down, try your own seasonings.

Prep time: **5 MINUTES**	Smoke time: **35 MINUTES**	Smoke temperature: **400°F**	Wood pellet flavor: **ALDER**

1 tablespoon olive oil

1 pound ground beef

1 (16-ounce) can kidney beans

1 (4-ounce) can diced green chiles

1 packet chili seasoning mix

14½ ounces water

1. Supply your smoker with wood pellets and follow the manufacturer's specific start-up procedure. Place a cast-iron skillet on the grill grate and preheat, with the lid closed, to 400°F.

2. Drizzle the skillet with the olive oil. Add the beef to the skillet and cook until the beef starts to brown, about 5 minutes, breaking up the beef into small pieces while cooking.

3. Once the beef is cooked, remove the skillet from the grill and drain off the grease. Return the skillet to the grill.

4. To the skillet, add the beans, chiles, seasoning mix, and water and combine.

5. Continue cooking for about 30 minutes, or until the liquid is absorbed, stirring occasionally.

6. Remove the skillet from the grill and serve.

Cooking tip: To add some smoke flavor, drop the grill to the smoke setting before all the liquid is absorbed in step 5. This will pack in some more wood-fire flavor, giving you all the more reason to cook your chili outside.

SLIGHTLY SMOKY, EASY, CHEESY MACARONI

Serves 6

If you are anything like me, you lived on macaroni and cheese as a kid. The best thing about getting older, along with being able to rent a car, is that our favorite dish from childhood no longer has to come from a cardboard box.

This is my version of mac and cheese. This recipe is simple enough, but it is spiked with some smoky flavor. Make this for your kiddos and kiss the boxed version goodbye.

Prep time: **5 MINUTES**	Smoke time: **30 MINUTES**	Smoke temperature: **400°F**	Wood pellet flavor: **COMPETITION BLEND**

16 ounces elbow macaroni

4 tablespoons (¼ cup) butter

¼ cup milk

4 ounces cream cheese, room temperature

4 ounces shredded mozzarella cheese

4 ounces shredded cheddar cheese

Kosher salt

Freshly ground black pepper

1. Supply your smoker with wood pellets and follow the manufacturer's specific start-up procedure. Place a deep cast-iron pot with a lid or a Dutch oven on the grill and preheat, with the grill lid closed, to 400°F.

2. In the pot, cook the pasta according to package directions. Drain and return the pasta to the pot.

3. Place the pot back on the grill grate and drop the grill to smoke or the lowest setting.

4. Stir in the butter and milk.

5. Add the cream cheese, mozzarella, cheddar, and salt and pepper, to taste, to the pasta. Stir well to combine.

6. Close the grill lid and smoke, pot uncovered, for 10 to 15 minutes.

7. Remove the pot from the grill and serve immediately.

Cooking tip: Put a thin layer of bread crumbs on top of your mac before smoking it in step 7, bringing home that home-cooked feel.

SMOKED GUACAMOLE

My family and I love guacamole. During our short time living in Phoenix, Arizona, it was our go-to snack. The price of avocados was significantly lower than in Oregon, and we took advantage of this. I have used the same method to create my guacamole for years. The combination of avocado, lime, and heat is perfect, and I don't like to mess with it.

Something that I have turned to doing in recent years is smoking my avocados before making my guacamole. A couple of years back I went to my friend Pat's house, where he served a barbecue feast that included smoked guacamole. He gave me tips on how to do it, and I took it from there.

Prep time:	Smoke time:	Smoke temperature:	Wood pellet flavor:
15 MINUTES	**20 MINUTES**	**180°F**	**HICKORY**

5 medium avocados

1 bunch fresh cilantro, stems trimmed and leaves finely chopped

1 tablespoon sour cream

1 teaspoon hot sauce (I use Tapatío)

Juice of 1 lime

1 teaspoon garlic powder

Kosher salt

Freshly ground black pepper

1. Supply your smoker with wood pellets and follow the manufacturer's specific start-up procedure. Preheat the grill, with the lid closed, to 180°F.

2. Slice the avocados in half and remove the seeds. Using a spoon, run it around the edge of the avocado half, separating the flesh from the peel. You want to keep the avocado half intact.

3. Set the avocado halves directly on the grill grate, cut-side down. Close the lid and smoke for about 20 minutes, or until the halves are soft and buttery.

4. Remove the avocados from the grill and place them into a large bowl. Add the cilantro, sour cream, hot sauce, lime juice, garlic powder, and salt and pepper to taste.

5. Lightly mash the mixture until smooth and serve with tortilla chips.

Cooking tip: I sometimes skip the sour cream in this recipe. Though I like the flavor it adds, you can easily make the guacamole without it to make it dairy-free, and omitting it will only have a slight effect on the final product.

GRILLED SUGAR CARROTS

I don't know whether to call this a side or a dessert. Grilled carrots are good on their own, but these will remind you of those buttery, sugary steamed ones you had as a kid.

The pellet grill gives us more freedom than any other outdoor cooker, which helps to make some of the better sides you will have. Adding wood-fired flavor to traditional meals is the best way to take your cooking over the top.

Prep time: **10 MINUTES**	Smoke time: **40 MINUTES**	Smoke temperature: **350°F**	Wood pellet flavor: **ALDER**

1½ pounds carrots, peeled and halved lengthwise

2 tablespoons olive oil

Kosher salt

Freshly ground black pepper

6 tablespoons butter, room temperature

4 tablespoons brown sugar

Cooking tip: Veggies are king on the pellet grill. Along with carrots, try grilling asparagus, zucchini, and other veggies.

1. Supply your smoker with wood pellets and follow the manufacturer's specific start-up procedure. Preheat the grill, with the lid closed, to 350°F.

2. Place the carrot halves in a large bowl and add the olive oil and salt and pepper to taste. Mix well, coating the carrots.

3. Place the carrots directly on the grill grate, close the lid, and cook for 20 minutes.

4. While the carrots cook, combine the butter and brown sugar in a small microwave-safe bowl, and microwave for about 25 seconds, stirring every 10 seconds.

5. After 20 minutes, use a basting brush to baste the carrots with the brown sugar butter. Flip and baste on the other side as well.

6. Cook for about 20 minutes more, or until the carrots are soft when pierced with a fork.

7. Remove the carrots from the grill and serve.

SWEET BAKED BEANS

Baked beans are another side where the pellet grill not only makes things easy but puts the flavor over the top. We all love baked beans with barbecue sauce, though this recipe adds a little something extra. My mom has perfected this side so well so that my oldest child has been known to ask for it about every other time we see them.

This is another quick recipe that uses a few items that you probably either already have or can pick up on your way home from work. Sweeten up your day with some smoky, sweet baked beans.

Prep time:	Smoke time:	Smoke temperature:	Wood pellet flavor:
3 MINUTES	**35 MINUTES**	**350°F AND 180°F**	**HICKORY**

1 (28-ounce) can baked beans (I use Bush's)

1 (8-ounce) can pineapple chunks, drained

Worcestershire sauce

¼ cup brown sugar

¼ cup ketchup

Freshly ground black pepper

Cooking tip: Use any of your favorite seasonings with this recipe. We love pepper in my house, but a Cajun or garlic seasoning also works great.

1. Supply your smoker with wood pellets and follow the manufacturer's specific start-up procedure. Place a deep cast-iron skillet with a lid or a Dutch oven onto the grill and preheat, with the lid closed, to 350°F.

2. In the skillet, combine the beans, pineapple chunks, 6 to 8 dashes Worcestershire sauce, the brown sugar, ketchup, and pepper to taste. Mix well and close the lid.

3. Bring to a soft boil and cook for about 30 minutes, or until the beans are warmed through. Reduce the temperature to 180°F and smoke for 5 minutes more.

4. Remove the skillet from the grill and serve immediately.

GRILLED POTATO WEDGES

Potato wedges are a classic side that takes next to no effort to cook. This treat is prepped in a matter of minutes by simply cutting up a few potatoes and covering them with oil and seasoning. This was something that I would have often growing up, and I still do. The wedges come off the grill tender, but slightly crunchy on the outside. The pellet grill completely cooks them while avoiding burning.

Prep time: **10 MINUTES**	Smoke time: **40 MINUTES**	Smoke temperature: **400°F**	Wood pellet flavor: **ALDER**

5 russet potatoes, washed

3 tablespoons olive oil

Rosemary-Garlic Seasoning (page 85)

1. Supply your smoker with wood pellets and follow the manufacturer's specific start-up procedure. Preheat the grill, with the lid closed, to 400°F.

2. Cut the potatoes into eighths, lengthwise, and place in a large bowl.

3. Add the olive oil and seasoning to taste, and mix well, ensuring the potatoes are coated evenly.

4. Place the potatoes on the grill grate, skin-side down. Close the lid and cook until soft, about 40 minutes.

5. Remove the potatoes and serve with ranch dressing, ketchup, or your favorite dipping sauce.

Cooking tip: Wedges are a cook that can easily be combined with another. At 400°F, 40 minutes gives us tons of options. Throw them on your top rack and cook up a steak or chicken breast on another rack. Cook the meat for the last 20 minutes of the wedges' cook time, and you have yourself a meal.

CAST-IRON POTATOES

Meat and potatoes are what many, myself included, think of when it comes to the perfect meal. By far, my favorite way to have potatoes is from a cast-iron skillet. After cutting up some small potatoes with onions and peppers, I cook them all up in the cast-iron skillet for perfect roasted potatoes.

Prep time: **15 MINUTES**	Smoke time: **20 MINUTES**	Smoke temperature: **400°F**	Wood pellet flavor: **HICKORY**

2 pounds baby red or yellow potatoes, washed and diced into bite-size chunks

3 tablespoons olive oil

½ white onion, diced

1 red bell pepper, cut into ½-inch pieces

Poultry Rub (page 84)

1. Supply your smoker with wood pellets and follow the manufacturer's specific start-up procedure. Place a cast-iron skillet onto the grill and preheat, with the lid closed, to 400°F.

2. Once the grill has reached temperature, pour the potatoes and olive oil into the skillet and mix well. Cook the potatoes, stirring occasionally, for about 15 minutes.

3. Once the potatoes are semisoft, add the onion and bell pepper and sprinkle with the rub to taste. Mix well and cook for about 5 minutes, or until the onion and pepper are softened.

4. Remove the potatoes from the grill and serve immediately.

Cooking tip: I recommend picking up a knife glove or two to help keep you from accidentally cutting yourself on meat, veggies, or anything else in the kitchen. I lost the tip of one of my fingers a few years back and now won't go without my knife glove.

CHEESY SCALLOPED POTATOES

My daughter Chloe loves scalloped potatoes. Her grandma and aunt make two of the best batches around, but we only get them around holidays. Earlier this year, Chloe bugged me to make them. After being disappointed with a couple of store-bought brands, I decided to give them a try myself, and I am sure glad I did.

After doing a little research online, I came up with an easy way to make the potatoes that also gave me the flavors I wanted. After a little trial and error, I made some of the best potatoes I have ever had, and they were a definite crowd-pleaser at the dinner table.

Prep time:	Smoke time:	Smoke temperature:	Wood pellet flavor:
15 MINUTES	**50 MINUTES**	**375°F**	**COMPETITION BLEND**

2 pounds russet potatoes, washed and thinly sliced into rounds

Kosher salt

Freshly ground black pepper

1 bunch fresh rosemary (finely chop the leaves from all but 2 or 3 sprigs), divided

Nonstick cooking spray

1 cup shredded cheddar cheese

½ cup shredded Parmesan cheese

2 cups heavy (whipping) cream

1. Supply your smoker with wood pellets and follow the manufacturer's specific start-up procedure. Preheat the grill, with the lid closed, to 375°F.

2. In a large bowl, toss together the potatoes, salt and pepper to taste, and the chopped rosemary to combine.

3. Grease a 13-by-9-inch pan and spread half the potatoes in an even layer on the bottom. Cover the potatoes with ½ cup cheddar and ¼ cup Parmesan cheese.

4. Layer on the remaining potatoes and top with the remaining ½ cup cheddar and ¼ cup Parmesan cheese, then pour the heavy cream over the cheese and potatoes evenly. Garnish with the remaining rosemary sprigs.

5. Place the pan on the grill grate, close the lid, and cook until the potatoes are soft, about 50 minutes.

6. Remove the potatoes from the grill and serve.

Cooking tip: Add sliced onions to your potatoes before cooking. I typically make this recipe without them to save me the tears, but many of the best scalloped potatoes I have had were full of onions.

CANDY BACON

I have always cooked my bacon on the grill. There are many ways to do it, from basic to extravagant. This recipe gives you an extravagant taste with little effort. Candy bacon, as the name implies, is a sweet and often seasoned bacon that is baked instead of fried. For this recipe, you will top the bacon with brown sugar and the Sweet Brown Sugar Rub for a perfectly salty, sweet treat.

Prep time: **5 MINUTES**	Smoke time: **2 HOURS**	Smoke temperature: **200°F**	Wood pellet flavor: **MAPLE**

1 (1-pound) package of thick-sliced pork bacon

½ cup brown sugar

Sweet Brown Sugar Rub (page 88)

1. Supply your smoker with wood pellets and follow the manufacturer's specific start-up procedure. Preheat the grill, with the lid closed, to 200°F.

2. Place the bacon slices directly on the grill grate, making sure they do not hang over the drain pan. Then sprinkle liberally with the brown sugar and the rub.

3. Close the grill lid and smoke the bacon to your preferred doneness.

4. Remove the bacon from the grill and serve immediately.

Cooking tip: A great way to cook bacon, with less of the mess, is to use a cookie rack/baking pan combo. Set the rack on top of the pan and the bacon on top of the rack. This allows the pan to collect the grease, keeping your drain pan clean.

SMOKED CHEESE

For this recipe, we are not even going to turn on the grill. By using a smoke tube, we can cold smoke cheese without the fear of it melting. Though I have smoked cheese with the grill running, there is a giant risk that the cheese will melt. In the dozens of times that I have smoked cheese, the most disappointing was when I walked out to a pool of cheese where there was once a block.

Prep time: **5 MINUTES**	Smoke time: **1 HOUR** **30 MINUTES** (plus overnight to chill)	Smoke temperature: **N/A**	Wood pellet flavor: **HICKORY**

1 (2-pound) block cheddar cheese

1. Supply your smoke tube with pellets and light using a torch or other method. Place inside the grill.

2. Slice the cheese into quarters, lengthwise, and place on a baking sheet.

3. Set the baking sheet on the grill grate, close the lid, and smoke until the smoke tube is completely out, about 1½ hours.

4. Remove the cheese from the grill and refrigerate overnight before serving.

Cooking tip: To help keep the inside of the grill cold and prevent melting, place a pan of ice under the grill grate, on the drain pan. The ice will work to keep the internal temperature of the grill down.

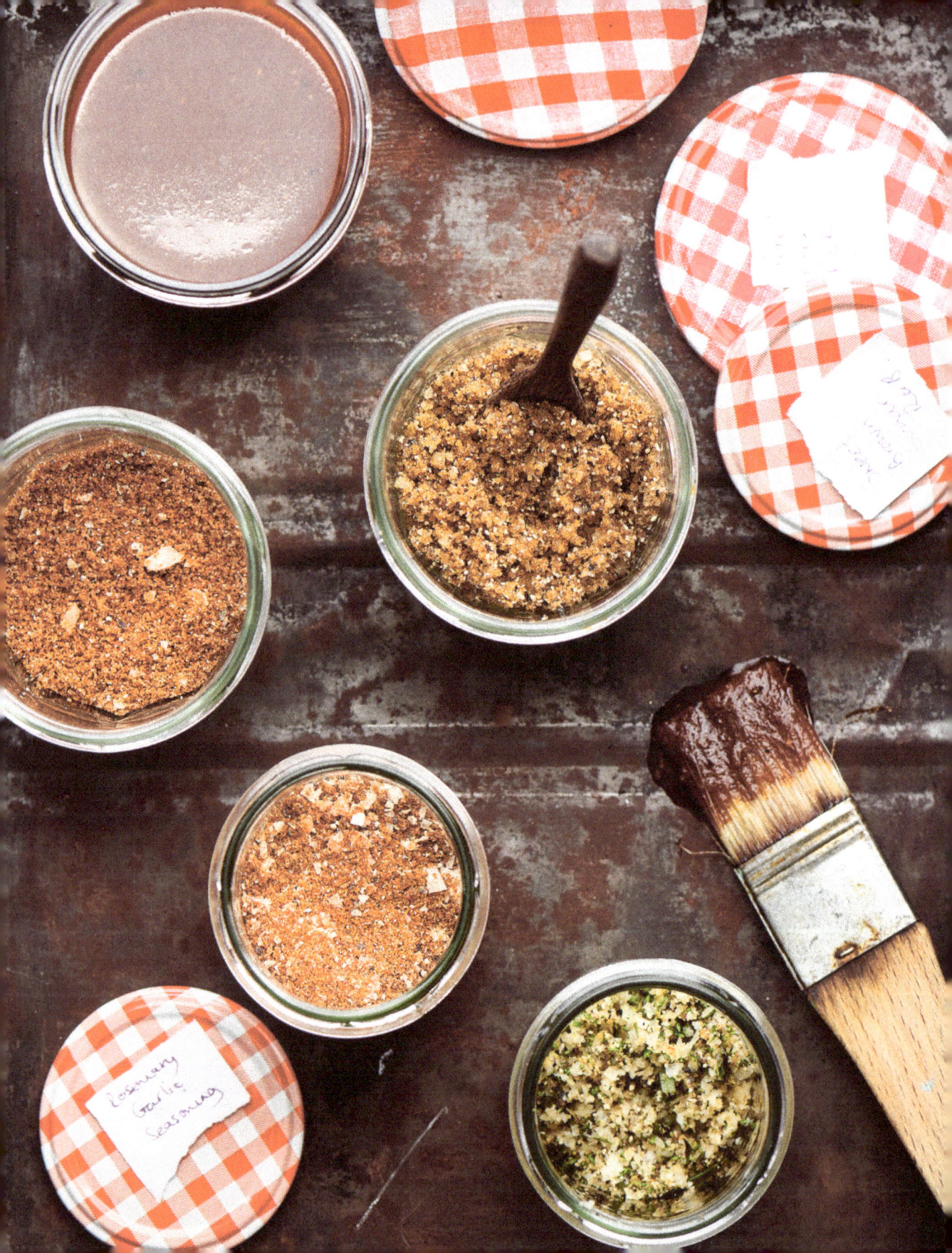

RUBS & SAUCES

BEEF AND BRISKET RUB

A basic beef and brisket rub is a grilling staple. Not only is this recipe made with few ingredients, but it has all the flavors you need to complement all cuts of beef. From brisket to prime rib, these simple ingredients will help bring together the natural flavors of the smoke and the meat.

Prep time:
5 MINUTES

3 tablespoons coarse kosher salt

1 tablespoon kosher salt

2 tablespoons freshly ground black pepper

1 tablespoon garlic powder

½ tablespoon onion powder

1. In a small bowl, mix together the coarse kosher salt, kosher salt, pepper, garlic powder, and onion powder.

2. Store any unused rub in a zip-top bag or airtight container. The rub can be stored for several months.

Cooking tip: I use sea salt instead of kosher salt in most of my rubs, but it comes with a major drawback. Sea salt sucks the moisture from whatever you use it on, kind of like your wood pellets, and any leftover seasoning tends to clump. As a rule of thumb, if I think there is a chance that I will have leftover rub, I opt for kosher salt.

PERFECT PORK RUB

A quality pork rub goes a long way. With so many different cuts, pork has a lot to offer, and you need great seasonings to complement it. I have played with many different ingredients to make the best possible rub for pork. This rub will not only give you the flavor to make your pork pop, but it is made from basic ingredients that you should have around the kitchen.

Prep time:
5 MINUTES

¼ **cup brown sugar**

1 **teaspoon coarse kosher salt**

1 **teaspoon garlic powder**

1 **teaspoon onion powder**

1 **teaspoon freshly ground black pepper**

1 **teaspoon paprika**

½ **teaspoon cayenne pepper**

¼ **teaspoon cinnamon**

1. In a small bowl, mix together the brown sugar, salt, garlic powder, onion powder, black pepper, paprika, cayenne pepper, and cinnamon.

2. Store any unused rub in a zip-top bag or air-tight container. The rub can be stored for several months.

Cooking tip: This pork rub can often double for a poultry rub. Compared to the Poultry Rub (page 84), this Perfect Pork Rub is far sweeter and can add that flavor to your chicken or turkey.

POULTRY RUB

Having a great poultry rub is an absolute necessity for me. At our home, chicken is something we almost always agree on, and this rub gives me quality flavors that will work well with all cuts of poultry, light or dark.

Prep time:
5 MINUTES

3 tablespoons kosher salt

2 tablespoons freshly ground black pepper

2 tablespoons brown sugar

1 tablespoon garlic powder

½ tablespoon onion powder

1 teaspoon cumin

1. In a small bowl, mix together the salt, pepper, brown sugar, garlic powder, onion powder, and cumin.

2. Store any unused rub in a zip-top bag or air-tight container. The rub can be stored for several months.

Cooking tip: When making rubs and sauces for your grill, only use all-natural sugars. Artificial sugars do not respond well to high heat and will not caramelize the way you want them to.

ROSEMARY-GARLIC SEASONING

I love the flavor of rosemary on just about everything. One of my favorite things to do for many of my dishes is to cut up some fresh rosemary and throw it in with the seasoning. I will oftentimes cook my steaks on a bed of rosemary or place a bunch inside my chicken or turkey.

For the times that I do not have fresh rosemary handy, I use this recipe, which gives you a great seasoning packed with that rosemary flavor.

Prep time:
5 MINUTES

---

3 teaspoons minced rosemary

3 teaspoons coarse kosher salt

1 teaspoon garlic powder

1 teaspoon freshly ground black pepper

½ teaspoon minced garlic

½ teaspoon minced onion

1. In a small bowl, mix together the rosemary, salt, garlic powder, pepper, minced garlic, and minced onion.

2. Store any unused rub in a zip-top bag or air-tight container. The rub can be stored for several months.

Cooking tip: Use this seasoning with lamb, beef, game, or poultry. Rub your chicken or turkey with this and then throw a rosemary sprig or two inside the bird.

SUPERB SEAFOOD RUB

Makes ¼ cup

Seafood is my favorite food to eat and likely my favorite to cook. There are different varieties, each interesting to cook. It doesn't hurt that I am craving whatever I am cooking the entire time.

When selecting the perfect spices for seafood, I once again try to keep it simple. I use citrus flavor profiles to pair with garlic and a family favorite: black pepper.

Prep time:
5 MINUTES

4 tablespoons kosher salt

2 tablespoons freshly ground black pepper

2 tablespoons lemon pepper

2 tablespoons garlic powder

2 teaspoons dried dill weed

1. In a small bowl, mix together the salt, black pepper, lemon pepper, garlic powder, and dill weed.

2. Store any unused rub in a zip-top bag or air-tight container. The rub can be stored for several months.

Cooking tip: Mix the seafood rub with a melted stick of butter for either a dipping sauce or to baste the seafood.

SPICY RUB

If you're like me, you like it hot! If this book was written to my taste, this is likely the only seasoning we would use. I love spicy flavors, and this recipe goes a long way to highlight them in a rub. This rub can be used for just about every cook. I use Spicy Rub for chicken, seafood, pork, anything. Like I said, I like it hot.

Prep time:
5 MINUTES

3 tablespoons coarse kosher salt

2 tablespoons freshly ground black pepper

1 tablespoon brown sugar

1 tablespoon garlic powder

1 tablespoon paprika

½ tablespoon cayenne pepper

½ tablespoon onion powder

1. In a small bowl, mix together the salt, black pepper, brown sugar, garlic powder, paprika, cayenne pepper, and onion powder.

2. Store any unused rub in a zip-top bag or airtight container. The rub can be stored for several months.

Cooking tip: My favorite way to use Spicy Rub is with my wings. Using this rub on wings, smoked for an hour or so, charred, and covered in wing sauce, I can never complain. Pass the blue cheese.

SWEET BROWN SUGAR RUB

Makes ¼ cup

I take advantage of this Sweet Brown Sugar Rub in this book a good amount. A sweet rub is great for poultry and pork. When barbecuing, I'm often cooking for a crowd and trying to cater to others' tastes. As a dad, I know this all too well. Kids are picky eaters, but one way to always win them over is with sweets, and this same premise can be transferred to the grill. Sweet rubs, especially with pork, are key for success.

Prep time:
5 MINUTES

¼ cup brown sugar

2 teaspoons coarse kosher salt

1 teaspoon garlic powder

1 teaspoon onion powder

1 teaspoon paprika

1 teaspoon freshly ground black pepper

½ teaspoon cayenne pepper

¼ teaspoon smoked paprika

1. In a small bowl, mix together the brown sugar, salt, garlic powder, onion powder, paprika, black pepper, cayenne pepper, and smoked paprika.

2. Store any unused rub in a zip-top bag or air-tight container. The rub can be stored for several months.

Cooking tip: I use this sweet rub in recipes like Candy Bacon (page 78) and Wood-Fired Pork Chops (page 29), but it can be used with almost any meat for a sweet treat.

CARNE ASADA MARINADE

When I first got out of college and had a little more time to grill, I used to marinate everything. Chicken and beef were my favorites, but pork often wound up in a marinade as well. My favorite has always been a carne asada–style marinade. I have been known to use this with just about everything, including burgers.

Prep time:
5 MINUTES

½ cup water

½ cup soy sauce

⅓ cup
Worcestershire sauce

¼ cup olive oil

Juice of 1 lime

½ bunch
cilantro, chopped

2 garlic cloves, minced

2 tablespoons
brown sugar

2 tablespoons freshly
ground black pepper

1. In a small bowl, mix together the water, soy sauce, Worcestershire sauce, olive oil, lime juice, cilantro, garlic, brown sugar, and pepper.

2. Store any unused marinade in an airtight container and refrigerate for up to 1 week.

Cooking tip: Marinating times really do not matter much. Even after about 20 minutes, your meat will retain some of that flavor. I recommend marinating for anywhere from 30 minutes to 24 hours.

HONEY BBQ SAUCE

Makes 2 cups

Barbecue sauce is a science. In my opinion, there are some really good sauces and some really bad sauces. I have seen sauces completely flop because they just didn't hit with customers, and those customers shared their poor experience.

My barbecue sauces are based on one original recipe. The reason for this is that it is good. I tweak the spices a bit, as needed, but typically add something to present a whole new flavor profile. In this recipe, it is honey. Any leftover barbecue sauce can be stored in the refrigerator in an airtight container for up to one week.

Prep time:
10 MINUTES

Cook time:
10 MINUTES

2 tablespoons olive oil

½ white onion, minced

1 (8-ounce) can tomato sauce

½ cup brown sugar

¼ cup white vinegar

¼ cup honey

1½ tablespoons Worcestershire sauce

2 teaspoons chili powder

¼ teaspoon dry mustard

2 teaspoons kosher salt

1 teaspoon freshly ground black pepper

1. In a medium saucepan on the stovetop over medium-high heat, heat the oil until shimmering. Add the onion and stir until it is tender and semi-translucent, about 1 minute.

2. Stir in the tomato sauce, brown sugar, vinegar, honey, Worcestershire sauce, chili powder, dry mustard, salt, and pepper, mixing thoroughly.

3. Heat until boiling, about 9 minutes, stirring constantly.

4. Remove the sauce from the stovetop and serve with your favorite cut of meat.

Cooking tip: This sauce is perfect for ribs. I love the way the honey complements the flavor of the pork.

SPICY BBQ SAUCE

My favorite barbecue sauces always have a bit of spice to them. I don't know if it is the flavor it adds or just that hot kick that I like. From Texas Spicy to Five Monkeys, my current go-to sauce, they all have a little heat. For this recipe, you will add that heat yourself for the perfect sauce. Any leftover sauce can be stored in the refrigerator in an airtight container for up to one week.

Prep time:
10 MINUTES

Cook time:
10 MINUTES

2 tablespoons olive oil

½ white onion, minced

1 (8-ounce) can tomato sauce

½ cup brown sugar

¼ cup white vinegar

1½ tablespoons Worcestershire sauce

2 tablespoons hot sauce (I use Tapatío)

3 teaspoons chili powder

¼ teaspoon dry mustard

2 teaspoons kosher salt

2 teaspoons freshly ground black pepper

1. In a medium saucepan on the stovetop over medium-high heat, heat the oil until shimmering. Add the onion and stir until it is tender and semi-translucent, about 1 minute.

2. Add the tomato sauce, brown sugar, vinegar, Worcestershire sauce, hot sauce, chili powder, dry mustard, salt, and pepper, mixing thoroughly.

3. Heat until boiling, about 9 minutes, stirring constantly.

4. Remove the sauce from the stovetop and serve with your favorite cut.

Cooking tip: Experiment with different hot sauces. Each hot sauce has a different flavor that it can bring to any recipe.

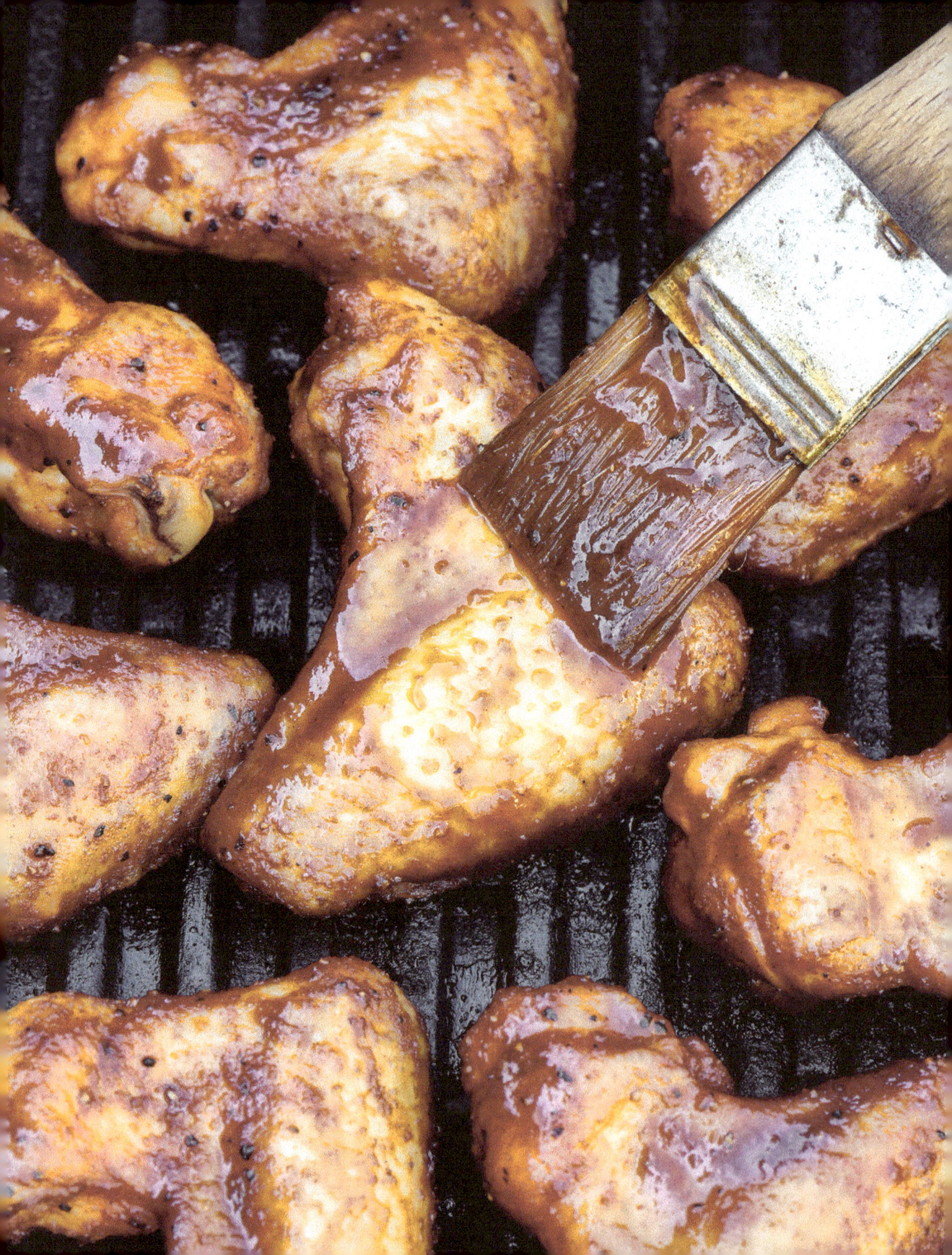

MEASUREMENT CONVERSIONS

VOLUME EQUIVALENTS	U.S. Standard	U.S. Standard (ounces)	Metric (approximate)
LIQUID	2 tablespoons	1 fl. oz.	30 mL
	¼ cup	2 fl. oz.	60 mL
	½ cup	4 fl. oz.	120 mL
	1 cup	8 fl. oz.	240 mL
	1½ cups	12 fl. oz.	355 mL
	2 cups or 1 pint	16 fl. oz.	475 mL
	4 cups or 1 quart	32 fl. oz.	1 L
	1 gallon	128 fl. oz.	4 L
DRY	⅛ teaspoon	—	0.5 mL
	¼ teaspoon	—	1 mL
	½ teaspoon	—	2 mL
	¾ teaspoon	—	4 mL
	1 teaspoon	—	5 mL
	1 tablespoon	—	15 mL
	¼ cup	—	59 mL
	⅓ cup	—	79 mL
	½ cup	—	118 mL
	⅔ cup	—	156 mL
	¾ cup	—	177 mL
	1 cup	—	235 mL
	2 cups or 1 pint	—	475 mL
	3 cups	—	700 mL
	4 cups or 1 quart	—	1 L
	½ gallon	—	2 L
	1 gallon	—	4 L

OVEN TEMPERATURES

Fahrenheit	Celsius (approximate)
250°F	120°C
300°F	150°C
325°F	165°C
350°F	180°C
375°F	190°C
400°F	200°C
425°F	220°C
450°F	230°C

WEIGHT EQUIVALENTS

U.S. Standard	Metric (approximate)
½ ounce	15 g
1 ounce	30 g
2 ounces	60 g
4 ounces	115 g
8 ounces	225 g
12 ounces	340 g
16 ounces or 1 pound	455 g

RESOURCES

Traeger Wood Pellet Grills

TraegerGrills.com/ Traeger makes the original wood pellet grill. Their site features not only their line of grills but also a huge collection of pellet grill recipes.

Pit Boss Grills

PitBoss-Grills.com/ Pit Boss is the second-largest pellet grill company and is quickly growing, with a diverse pellet grill and vertical smoker line. Visit the Pit Boss site for great pellet grill–related blog posts and educational videos.

Weber Grills

Weber.com/ Weber, the world's largest grill distributor, jumped onto the pellet grill bandwagon in 2020. Though they are new to pellet grills, Weber has a vast array of barbecue resources for grillers of all skill levels.

The BBQ Central Show

TheBBQCentralShow.com/ Best barbecue podcast you will find. Greg Rempe does an amazing job, has awesome guests, and talks pellet grills from time to time.

Master the Wood Pellet Grill by Andrew Koster

My first but most advanced pellet grill cookbook. When you are ready to step up your smoking game, grab this book for a plethora of pellet grill knowledge.

The Ultimate Wood Pellet Grill Smoker Cookbook by Bill West

Cookbook with collection of pellet grill tips, tricks, and recipes.

Flavor Train—Chuck Matto

TheFlavorTrain.com/ Chuck is a barbecue genius, and he spends most of his time with pellet grills. I get tons of my barbecue ideas from his Instagram page, @chucksflavortrain.

Cheeky BBQ—Noah Cheek

CheekyBBQ.com/ Noah is extremely knowledgeable in the pellet grill game. He knows tons about meat and how it is prepared.

Franklin BBQ—Aaron Franklin

FranklinBBQ.com/ Aaron Franklin is the king of Texas barbecue. You won't find anything specific to pellet grills, but he has tons of great information on barbecue and meat prep.

Five Monkeys BBQ Sauce

FiveMonkeysBBQSauce.com/ In my opinion, the best barbecue sauce on the market.

Louisiana Outdoor Cooking by Jay Ducote

Jay Ducote is a Food Network star and, in my humble opinion, the king of Louisiana barbecue. Jay has made multiple appearances on ESPN's *College GameDay*, and he shares much of his tailgate knowledge in his book *Louisiana Outdoor Cooking*.

Petromax

Petromax.de/en/ I use Petromax cast iron. It is pre-seasoned and high quality. The brand only recently became available in the United States.

FireBoard

FireBoard.com/ FireBoard is a third-party thermometer. It uses both Wi-Fi and Bluetooth to communicate your grill and meat temperatures to your Android or iPhone, via an app.

A-MAZE-N

AMAZENProducts.com/ A-MAZE-N smoke tubes are awesome to use for aid in smoke production as well as in place of a cold smoker.

INDEX

ACKNOWLEDGMENTS

I would like to thank anyone who has given me an opportunity in barbecue. First and foremost, my dad, George Koster. Dan, Jeff, and Jordan Thiessen, Joe Traeger, and Keith Barish have all given me opportunities to learn and grow in the pellet grill world.

My family has always been in my corner, and I could do none of this without Chanelle, Brianna, Chloe, and Andrew's support and help. Mom, Dad, Brooke, and Cody, thanks for always being there.

ABOUT THE AUTHOR

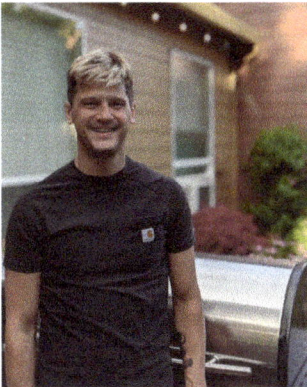

Andrew Koster is among the world's foremost experts on pellet grills. He is the author of *Master the Wood Pellet Grill: A Cookbook to Smoke Meats Like a Pro* as well as the former customer service manager of Traeger, Pit Boss, and Louisiana Grills. On top of helping countless customers learn and conquer the pellet grill, Andrew has also assisted in the development of multiple pellet grills, including the Traeger Timberline and Pit Boss Platinum and Pro Series as well as Louisiana Grills Black Label and Founders Series.

Andrew currently works as a member of the research and development team at Dansons, the maker of Pit Boss and Louisiana Grills, and lives in Silverton, Oregon, with his wife, Chanelle, and his three children, Brianna, Chloe, and Andrew Jr.

CPSIA information can be obtained
at www.ICGtesting.com
Printed in the USA
JSHW051908180722
28015JS00006B/6